Traditional Chinese Treatment for Respiratory Diseases

Chief－Editor: Hou Jinglun　Zhou Xunmei
Editor: Zhao Xin、Luo Guohua　Geng Chun'e

Academy Press [Xue Yuan]

First Edition 1996
ISBN7－5077－1205－2/R・215

Traditional Chinese Treatment for Respiratory Diseases
Chief－Editor: Hou Jinglun Zhou Xunmei
Editor: Zhao Xin Luo Guohua Geng Chun'e

Published by
Academy Press [Xue Yuan]
11 Wanshoulu Xijie, Beijing 100036, China

Distributed by
China International Book Trading Corporation
35 Chegongzhuang Xilu, Beijing 100044, China
P. O. Box 399, Beijing, China

Printed in the People's Republic of China

Preface

Traditional Chinese Medicine and Pharmacology(TCMP) has a long history. It summed up abundant clinical experience in the struggle against diseases. It has formed an integrated, unique and first of all, a scientific system of both theory and clinical practice. On the fundamental principle of Zhengtiguannian (Wholism) and Bianzhenglunzhi (Treatment of the same disease with different therapies). TCM treatment is effective for various kinds of diseases with few side—effect taken. At present, a great upsurge in learning, practising and studying TCM is just in the ascendant.

In this book, we introduced comprehensively TCM treatment for commonly encountered diseases of the respiratory system and therapies such as drug therapy, acupuncture and moxibustion, Qigong, massage, dietic therapy, etc. are suggested accordingly. This book is the best for those foreign friends who want to learn and master traditional Chinese medicine.

May everyone of all nations enjoy a healthy life!

Chief—Editor

CONTENTS

Chapter One
Cough

Cough is a common disease, which occurs in all four seasons, especially in winter and spring. The incidence is high in babies under three years of age. The younger the cases are, the more severe the pathological conditions will be. Cough is often caused by invasion of external pathogenic factors, its duration short and its prognosis good.

When lung and defensive qi are weak, the external pathogenic wind－cold or wind－heat is likely to invade the lung system via the mouth, nose and skin pores, thus impairing the function of the lung in dispersing and descending. Subsequently, cough will result. Retention of phlegm－damp in the spleen and lung can also cause cough when induced by invasion of external pathogenic factors.

ETIOLOGY AND PATHOGENESIS

1. **Cough attacked by exogenous pathogenic factors.** When weather is changeable in winter and spring, six exogenous pathogenic factors will easily attack the lung, resulting in cough due to impairment of purifying and descending function of the lung and abnormal rising of lung－qi. As the result of the sluggishness of lung－qi, the interior retention and accumulation of the body fluid will form sputum, obstructing the air passage and inducing productive cough.

2. **Stagnation of phlegm in the interior**. The stagnation of dampness may be transformed into sputum which will store in the lung, block the air passage and inhibit ventilation.

3. **Weak constitution**. People are apt to be invaded by exogenous pathogenic factors if they are congenitally deficient and weak in constitution. The invasion brings about recurrent cough. Chronic cough will injure the spleen and the lung and result in cough by the internal injury due to deficiency of both the spleen and the lung, and the consumption of the lung－yin.

MAIN POINTS OF DIAGNOSIS

1. The initial onset of the cough caused by exogenous pathogenic factors is mostly accompanied by cold symptoms such as chilliness, fever, stuffy nose with watery discharge, headache, general muscular pains, redness and itching of the throat. After one or two

days, it is chiefly marked by cough. At first, the cough may present with deep, loud or raucous sound, which is mild during the day and severe at night, associated with vomiting, and thin whitish or thick yellowish sputum. However, young children are unable to spit.

2. Cough caused by internal injury is commonly seen in the cases with delicate constitution and malnutrition. These people are likely to catch a cold and will be more severely attacked by pathogenic factors. The course of the disease is rather long, manifested by cough low cough with thin whitish or less thick sputum or associated with fever.

DIFFERENTIATION AND TREATMENT OF COMMON SYNDROMES

Acute cough is due to the affection of exopathogen, usually accompanied with exterior syndrome. The treatment is mainly to dispel the pathogenic factor attacking the exterior of the body and ventilate the lung to relieve cough. Chronic cough is mostly classified deficiency syndrome caused by internal injury. The treatment is mainly to strengthen the body resistance to resolve phlegm and astringing the lung to relieve cough.

1. Cough caused by the affection of exopathogen

1) Cough due to pathogenic wind - cold

Main Symptoms and Signs: Recurrent cough with heavy sound, itching feeling of the throat, difficultly expectorated sputum or cough with rale, thin and whitish sputum, chilliness, fever, stuffy nose with watery discharge, headache and pantalgia, thin and whitish fur on the tongue, and floating and tense pulse.

This syndrome is due to invasion of the lung by external pathogenic wind - cold, which impairs the lung's function in dispersing and descending. Since the lung opens into the nose, nasal obstruction with clear discharge and choking cough result. The invasion of the body surface by wind - cold does not allow the skin pores to open and close normally, thus giving rise to such symptoms as fever, aversion to cold and absence of sweating.

Therapeutic Principles: Expelling wind and cold pathogens, and ventilating the lung and relieving cough.

Recipe: Xing su san (Powder of apricot kernel and perilla), modified.

Folium Perillae	6 g
Semen Armenicacae Amerum	3 g
Radix Peucedani	9 g
Radix Platycodi	9 g
Herba Schizonepetae	9 g

Rhizoma Pinelliae 9 g
Fructus Aurantii 6 g
Radix Glycyrrhizae 3 g

All the above drugs are to be decocted in water for oral administration.

Modification: If the exterior syndrome is more severe associated with severe and unsmooth cough, *Radix Ledebouriellae* 9 g and *Herba Ephedrae* 6 g should be added to relieve exterior syndrome and ventilate the lung. If exterior syndrome has been relieved, and only cough is marked, *Radix Asteris* 9 g, *Flos Farfarae* 6 g and *Radix Stemonae* 9 g should be added or Zhi sou san be used to warm the lung, regulate the flow of qi and arrest cough.

2) **Cough due to pathogenic wind – heat**

Main Symptoms and Signs: It is manifested by cough with yellowish sputum too ropy to be expectorated, thirst, red and swelling throat with pain, fever with aversion to wind, slight sweat, turbid nasal discharge, red tip of the tongue with yellowish fur, and floating and rapid pulse.

This syndrome is due to invasion of the lung by external pathogenic heat. Retention of heat in the lung is the cause of cough in coarse or hoarse voice. Consumption of the fluid of the lung results in thick and yellow stomach, redness and soreness of the throat is the consequence of invasion of the lung and stomach by wind – heat. A red tongue with thin and yellow coating and a superficial and rapid pulse are both signs of wind – heat.

Therapeutic Principles: Dispelling wind, clearing away heat, ventilating the lung and resolving phlegm.

Recipe: Sāng ju yin (Decoction of Mulberry leaf and Chrysanthemum), modified.

Folium Mori 6 g
Flos Chrysanthemi 9 g
Herba Menthae 6 g
Semen Armeniacae Amarum 6 g
Radix Platycodi 9 g
Rhizoma Phragmitis 9 g
Fructus Forsythiae 12 g
Bulbus Fritillariae Thunbergii 6 g
Radix Scutellariae 9 g

All the above drugs are to be decocted in water for oral administration.

Modification: In case of severe fever with swelling and painful throat, *Fructus Gardeniae* 6 g and *Radix Isatidis* 12 g are added to relieve sore – throat and subdue swelling; if manifested by productive cough, thirst, irritability, and yellowish and greasy fur on the tongue, *Cortex Mori Radicis* 9 g, *Rhizoma Pinelliae* 9 g and *Poria* 9 g be added to expel wind and heat, ventilate the lung and remove dampness.

3) Cough due to wind – dryness

Main Symptoms and Signs: Cough with hoarseness, dry cough or cough with less sputum which is difficult to expectorate, dry lips, dryness and itching of throat, red tongue with less fur, shortness of saliva, and rapid pulse.

Therapeutic Principles: Promoting the dispersing function of the lung with drugs of acrid taste and cool nature, clearing away the lung – heat and moisturizing the lung.

Recipe: Sang xing tang (Decoction of Mulberry leat and Apricot kernel)

Folium Mori	9 g
Semen Armeniacae Amarum	6 g
Bulbus Fritillariae Thunbergii	6 g
Fructus Gardeniae	6 g
Radix Adenophorae Strictae	9 g
Exocarpium Pyrus	9 g
Radix Platycodi	9 g
Radix Scrophulariae	9 g

All the above drugs are to be decocted in water for oral administration.

2. Cough caused by internal injury

1) Cough due to phlegm and heat

Main Symptoms and Signs: Cough with abundant yellowish and thick expectoration, fever with flushed face and red lips, thirst, restlessness or epistaxis, dry stool, dark urine, red tongue with yellowish fur, and slippery and rapid pulse.

Therapeutic Principles: Clearing away heat and purging fire, and resolving phlegm and relieving cough.

Recipe: Xie bai san (Lung – heat expelling powder), modified.

Cortex Mori Radicis	9 g
Cortex Lycii Radicis	12 g
Radix Platycodi	9 g
Bulbus Fritillariae Cirrhosae	6 g
Radix Scutellariae	9 g
Semen Lepidii seu Descurainiae	6 g
Semen Plantaginis	9 g
Radix Glycyrrhizae	3 g

All the above drugs are to be decocted in water for oral administration.

Modification: If it is manifested by cough with sputum too thick to be expectorated,

Fructus Trichosanthis 9 g, *Os Costaziae* 12 g and *Arisaema cum Bile* 9 g should be added to remove heat – phlegm; if marked by constipation, overabundance of heat and harsh breath, *Semen Arecae* 9 g, *Fructus Aurantii Immaturus* 9 g and *Radix et Rhizoma Rhei* 6 g be added to remove the pathogenic fire from the lung.

2) **Cough due to phlegm – dampness**

Main Symptoms and Signs: Cough with whitish, thin and productive sputum, rale in the larynx, loss of appetite, listlessness, pale complexion, whitish and greasy fur on the pale tongue, and smooth pulse.

This syndrome is due to weakness of the spleen and lung, which allows frequent invasion by external pathogenic wind. This explains lingering cough. Deficiency of spleen qi results in pale complexion. Dysfunction of the spleen in transportation and transformation produces phlegm – damp, which is stored in the lung after being produced. Therefore, profuse sputum is the distinguishable symptom of this syndrome. A pale tongue with white, slippery and sticky coating, and a rolling pulse, are both signs of phlegm – damp.

Therapeutic Principles: Invigorating the spleen to dry the dampness, and resolving phlegm to relieve cough.

Recipe: Er chen tang (Two old drugs decoction), modified.

Pericarpium Citri Reticulatae	9 g
Rhizoma Pinelliae	9 g
Poria	9 g
Semen Armeniacae Amarum	6 g
Radix Platycodi	9 g
Bulbus Fritillariae Cirrhosae	6 g
Fructus Aurantii	9 g
Semen Raphani	9 g
Fructus Perillae	9 g
Radix Glycyrrhizae	3 g

All the above drugs are to be decocted in water for oral administration.

Modification: If there exists deficiency of spleen due to chronic cough, *Rhizoma Atractylodis Macrocephalae* 9 g and *Radix Codonopsis Pilosulae* 9 g should be added to invigorate the spleen. If associated with poor appetite and abdominal distention. *Massa Fermentata Medicinalis* 6 g, *Fructus Crataegi* 9 g and *Semen Raphani Praeparata* 9 g should be added to promote digestion and remove stagnated food.

3) **Cough due to yin deficiency**

Main Symptoms and Signs: Dry cough, or cough with less viscid or blood – tinged sputum, dryness in the mouth and throat, flushed cheeks, fever with night sweat, feverish sensation in the palms and soles, red and dry tongue with less fur, and fine and rapid pulse.

Therapeutic Principle: Nourishing yin and moisturizing the lung.

Recipe: Shashen maidong tang (Decoction of Adenophorae Strictae and Ophiopogonis), modified.

Radix Adenophorae Strictae	12 g
Radix Ophiopogonis	9 g
Rhizoma Polygonati Odorati	9 g
Radix Trichosanthis	9 g
Bulbus Fritillariae Thunbergii	6 g
Folium Eriobotryae Praeparata	9 g
Semen Dolichoris Alba	9 g
Radix Glycyrrhizae	3 g

All the above drugs are to be decocted in water for oral administration.

Modification: If it is accompanied with blood – stained sputum, *Rhizoma Bletillae* 9 g, *Rhizoma Imperatae* 12 g, *Colla Corii Asini* 9 g (melted) and *Radix Rehmanniae* 9 g should be added to moisturize the lung and stop bleeding, if it presents with hectic fever and night sweat, *Herba Artemisiae Chinghao* 12 g, *Cortex Lycii Radicis* 12 g and *Carapax Trionycis* 12 g should be added to nourish yin and clear away heat.

4) **Chronic cough due to deficiency of lung – yin**

Main Symptoms and Signs: Weak cough with whitish, thin and clear sputum, pale complexion, hyperidrosis due to general deficiency of qi, weak voice with no inclination to talk, lassitude and intolerance of cold, pale tender tongue, and fine and weak pulse.

Therapeutic Principles: Strengthening the spleen and replenishing qi.

Recipe: Liu junzi tang (Decoction of six ingredients), modified.

Radix Pseudostellariae	12 g
Poria	9 g
Rhizoma Atractylodis Macrocephalae	9 g
Rhizoma Pinelliae	9 g
Fructus Schisandrae	6 g
Radix Astragali seu Hedysari	9 g
Radix Platycodi	9 g
Radix Glycyrrhizae	3 g

All the above drugs are to be decocted in water for oral administration.

OTHER THERAPIES

1. simple recipe and proved prescription

1) *Fructus Perillae* 9 g, *Pericarpium Citri Reticulatae* 9 g and *raddish* (*in pieces*) 12 g, together with some *brown sugar* are all decocted in water for oral dose, which is applicable to cough due to wind – cold syndrome.

2) *Bulbus Fritillariae Cirrhosae* 6 g, *pear* (one without the core) and *crystal sugar* 15 g are decocted in water, or steamed for oral administration, which is suitable for dry cough.

3) Zhi ke san: *Bulbus fritillariae Cirrhosae*, *Semen Lepidii seu Descurainiae* and *Rhizoma Pinelliae*, all of equal portions, are made into rough powder, which is suitable for cough due to phlegm – heat. When taking, decoct the above ingredients in a small amount of water over soft fire for 2 – 3 minutes for oral dose, 3 times daily.

2. Acupuncture treatment

1) Body acupuncture

(1) **Excess syndromes**

Therapeutic Principles: To promote the lung's function in dispersing and relieve exterior symptoms. Points are mainly selected from the Lung and Urinary Bladder Meridians, and are needled with reducing method. Moxibustion is also applied to the points on the back in case of cold syndromes.

Prescription: Fengmen(BL12), Feishu(BL13), Chize(LU5), Lieque(LU7).

Explanation: Fengmen (BL12), the gateway of pathogenic wind, and Feishu (BL13), the Back – Shu Point of the lung, both act to eliminate wind and promote the lung's function in dispersing. Chize(LU5) and Lieque(LU7) relieve exterior symptoms and check coughing. In case of fever, Dazhui(DU14), Quchi(LI11) and Hegu(LI4) added. Add Yingxiang(LI20) and Shangxing(DU23) in case of nasal discharge. Add Fenglong(ST40) for phlegm.

(2) **Deficiency syndrome (phlegm – damp)**

Therapeutic Principles: To invigorate the spleen, resolve damp, eliminate phlegm and check coughing. Points are mainly selected from the Urinary Bladder and Stomach Meridians, and are needled with even method.

Prescription: Pishu(BL20), Feishu(BL13), Zusanli(ST36), Fenglong(ST40).

Explanation: Feishu(BL20) promotes the lung's function of dispersing and checks coughing. Pishu(BL20), Zusanli(ST36) and Fenglong(ST40) invigorate the spleen and resolve phlegm. Add Neiguan(PC6) and Danzhong(RN17) for stuffiness in the chest and difficulty in expectorating sputum.

2) **Auricular acupuncture**

Points: Fei(CO14) lung, Shenmen(TF4) shenmen, Qiguan(CO16) trachea, Neibi (TG4) internal nose.

Method: These points are needled bilaterally with equal stimulation.

Needles are not retained. Treatment is given every other day. Or rape seeds are implanted on ear points and renewed every three days.

Add Pi(CO13) spleen, Dachang(CO7) large intestine and Jiaogan(AH6a) sympathesis in case of profuse sputum due to deficiency of the spleen.

3) Tapping with plum - blossom needle

Points: Fengmen(BL12), Feishu(BL12), the Lung Meridian and the meridians passing through the arm.

Method: Each area is tapped with moderate stimulation for 3 - 5 minutes until the skin becomes red.

PREVENTION AND NURSING

1. Do more physical exercise to reinforce the body resistance against diseases.

2. Pay attention to weather changes and the prevention of cold. For those who have cough due to recurrent respiratory infection, care of the lung should be emphasized, cold aerotherapy and warm sponge are helpful to enhance resistance against diseases.

3. Keep the patient's room quiet with fresh flowing air to avoid cross infection.

DISCUSSION

Cough discussed in this section corresponds to acute bronchitis. Attention should be paid to the duration of the disease, coughing sound and sputum, in differentiation. Cough due to invasion by external pathogenic factors is often of short duration, while cough due to injury of internal organs is of long duration. Choking cough in strong voice is due to invasion of the lung by wind - cold; cough in coarse or hoarse voice is due to invasion of the lung by wind - heat; and fits of dry cough with shortness of the breath is due to retention of phlegm - heat in the lung. Thin and white sputum indicates cold; thick and yellow sputum indicates heat; and large amounts of thin and frothy sputum which can be easily expectorated indicate retention of phlegm and fluid. Patients should rest well, refrain from oily food, and take care not to be exposed to cold, especially the chest and back. Proper exercises are necessary in order to strengthen body resistance when the disease is resolved.

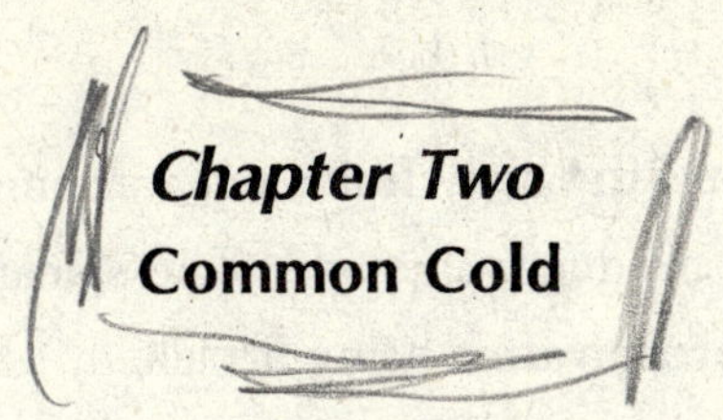

Chapter Two
Common Cold

Common cold is one of the most common diseases, and is characterized by fever, aversion to cold, nasal obstruction, runny nose, sneezing, coughing and headache. This disease can occur in all four seasons, but more commonly in winter and spring when there is a drastic change in weather, and in cases of all ages. The younger the patients are, the more the complications there will be. This is the principal characteristic of the common cold of children, which does not appear in adults.

ETIOLOGY AND PATHOGENESIS

Pathogenic wind is the predominant etiological factor in colds. It invades the upper respiratory tract and the body surface when body resistance is low, which typically occurs when there is a sudden climatic change. The pathogenic wind combines with cold in winter, heat in spring and damp – heat in summer, taking advantage of untimely climatic changes to attack the body.

The attack on the body is closely related to body resistance, so if one's vital energy is low due to an irregular life style, drenching by rain, negligence regarding changes in temperature or overfatigue, the likelihood of invasion increases. A patient with chronic bronchitis or bronchiectasis is also vulnerable. Furthermore, the body's constitution plays a role in the affection. A person with a yang deficiency is susceptible to wind – cold, and one with a yin deficiency is susceptible to wind – heat.

Because pathogenic wind invades through the upper respiratory tract and the body surface, pathological changes are confined to these portions of the body. When pathogenic factors obstruct the upper respiratory tract, respiratory symptoms occur, such as cough and stuffy nose. The confrontation between the body's resistance and pathogenic factors at the superficial portion of the body results in chilliness and fever.

In case of Delicate visceral organs, thin skin and weak Wei – system in combination with sudden change of the weather, the six exopathogenic factors are apt to attack the superficies to cause failure of superficial qi, disorder of opening and closing function of skin striae and inhibition of yang energy, manifested by fever and chills, headache, running and stuffy nose, cough etc.

In young cases of common cold, fever may be severe. It is because young children are of pure yang bodies and the invasion of evils is liable to bring about heat. Because of the delicate lungs in young cases, when they are attacked by evils, the lung – qi will stagnate, and qi will be out of order, and the body fluids may accumulate to form sputum, obstructing the air passages, causing productive cough. The spleen of young cases is not fully developed. If their diet is not proper after being attacked, the digestive function may be involved, milk and food may stagnate in the middle – jiao. They may present with distention of gastric cavity and abdomen, poor appetite for milk and food, vomiting or diarrhea, and some other dyspeptic symptoms. The invasion of evils will cause heat and fire, affecting the spirit, leading to vigilance and restlessness, even infantile convulsion. This is known as cold with convulsion in pediatrics.

MAIN POINTS OF DIAGNOSIS

1. **Main Symptoms and Signs**: It is mostly manifested by sudden onset, fever with no or little sweat, running and stuffy nose, sore throat, mild cough, etc. The body temperature is varied with different strains of pathogen type of disease and individual condition. Infants and younger children tend to have higher temperature than the older ones, sometimes reaching 40℃, but with better general condition. Older children have more severe localized symptoms of the nose, pharynx and throat.

2. **Complications**: In infants and young children, it is usually associated with high fever, convulsion or vomiting, diarrhea, abdominal pain, anorexia or productive cough, and even bronchitis or pneumonia.

3. Some acute infectious diseases such as measles, chicken pox, scarlet fever, epidemic mumps, epidemic encephalomyelitis, etc. have the same manifestations as colds in their early stages, but different features will soon be found later. So early identification is very necessary.

DIFFERENTIATION AND TREATMENT OF COMMON SYNDROMES

1. Common cold of wind – type

Main Symptoms and Signs: It is characterized by light fever, chilliness with no sweat, headache, cold nose with watery discharge, sneezing, mild cough, itching of the throat, thin and whitish fur on the tongue, and floating and tense pulse.

Invasion of the body surface by wind – cold leads to the conflict between the pathogenic factors and body resistance, and thereby produces fever and aversion to cold. The closing of the pores is the cause of absence of sweating. Dysfunction of lung qi in dispersing results in nasal obstruction with clear discharge and coughing. Since cold has not yet transformed into heat, there is absence of inflamed throat and thirst. A white tongue coating, a superficial and tense pulse, and a superficial and red capillary vessel are all signs of wind – cold.

Therapeutic Principles: Dispelling the evil in the superficies with drugs of acrid taste and warm nature and releasing stagnated lung – qi and cold.

Recipe: *Jing fang bai du san* (*Antiphlogistic powder of Schizonepeta and Ledebouriella*)

Herba Schizonepetae 6 g
Radix Ledebouriellae 6 g
Folium Perillae 6 g
Rhizoma seu Radix Notopterygii 9 g
Radix Bupleuri 12 g
Radix Platycodi 9 g
Radix Glycyrrhizae 3 g

Decoct the above ingredients in a right amount of water for oral administration.

Modification: In case of high fever, gneral disturbance and thirst, *Jiajian chai ge jie ji tang* is applicable. The recipe comprises:

Radix Bupleuri 15 g
Radix Puerariae 12 g
Gypsum Fibrosum 18 g
Radix Rehmanniae 9 g
Flos Lonicerae 12 g
Fructus Forsythiae 12 g
Herba Menthae 6 g
Folium Isatidis 9 g
Rhizoma Phragmitis 9 g
Radix Glycyrrhizae 3 g

Decoct the above ingredients in a right amount of water for oral administration.

If high fever is accompanied with convulsion, *Ramulus Uncariae cum Uncis* 6 g, *Bombyx Batryticatus* 9 g and *Periostracum Cicadae* 6 g should be added to calm the liver, relieve the convulsion and inhibit the wind – evil. If constipation is present, *Fructus Aurantii Immaturus* 9 g and *Fructus Trichosanthis* 9 g should be added to eliminate the fire by purgation.

3. Cold of summer – heat type

Main Symptoms and Signs: It is marked by high fever with no sweat, headache, heavy sensation of the body, listlessness, poor appetite or vomiting and diarrhea, running or stuffy nose, red tongue with thin whitish and slightly greasy fur, and floating and rapid pulse.

Therapeutic Principles: Clearing summer – heat evil and expelling superficial evils, and eliminating the dampness – evil and regulating stomach – qi.

Recipe: *Xiangru yin* (*Decoction of Elsholtzia with Supplements*), modified.

Herba Elsholtziae seu Moslae 9 g
Cortex Magnoliae Officinalis 9 g
Flos Dolichoris 9 g
Flos Lonicerae 12 g
Fructus Forsythiae 9 g
Herba Lophatheri 6 g
Radix Puerariae 9 g
Radix Glycyrrhizae 3 g

Decoct the above ingredients in a right amount of water for oral administration.

Modification: In case of light summer – heat but severe wetness – evil syndrome, manifested by headache, dizziness, feeling of fullness and oppression over the chest and abdomen, poor appetite, etc., *Herba Agastachis* 12 g, *Folium Perillae* 9 g, *Cortex Magnodiae Officinalis* 9 g, *Rhizoma Pinelliae* 9 g, *Pericarpium Citri Reticulatae* 6 g and *Rhizoma Atractylodis Macrocephalae* 9 g should be added to dispel the wetness – evil and regulate the stomach – qi. In case of severe summer – heat syndrome, marked by vexation, thirst, vomiting, less urine and failure of perspiration, etc., *Rhizoma coptidis* 3 g, *Herba Lophatheri* 6 g, *Rhizoma Phragmitis* 12 g and *Talcum* 9 g should be added to clear away summer – heat.

4. Cold of Autumn Dryness

Main Symptoms and Signs: It is characterized by fever with flushed face, no sweat, headache, dry stuffy nose, dry throat, cough without sputum or with sputum containing blood, red tongue with less dry fur, and small pulse.

Therapeutic Principles: Clearing away heat – evil with drugs of acrid taste and cool nature and moisturizing dryness – syndrome to relieve the cough.

Recipe: *Sang xing tang* (*Decoction of Mulberry leaf and Apricot kernel*), modified.

Folium Mori 6 g
Fructus Gardeniae 3 g
Semen Armeniacae Amarum 4.5 g
Bulbus Fritillariae Thunbergii 6 g
Radix Adenophorae Strictae 12 g
Exocarpium Pyrus 9 g
Gypsum Fibrosum 18 g

Radix Ophiopogonis	9 g
Colla Cori Asini	6 g
Radix Glycyrrhizae	3 g

Decoct the above ingredients in a right amount of water for oral administration.

Modification: In case of chronic cough, *Radix Stemonae Praeparata* 9 g, *Cortex Lycii Radicis* 12 g, *Fructus Schisandrae* 6 g and *Fructus Chebulae* 9 g should be added to relieve cough by astringing the liver. In case of long – standing low fever, dry skin, sputum containing blood, feverish sensation over the palms and soles, dizziness and feeling of distention in the eyes, the recipe, Shashen maidong tang should be applied by adding *Radix Rehmanniae* 12 g, *Cortex Moutan Radicis* 9 g, *Fructus Gardeniae* 4.5 g, and *Radix Scrophulariae* 9 g to nourish yin and clear away heat evil. If the patient reveals hoarse voice, *Radix Ophiopogonis* 9 g, *Radix Isalidis* 12 g, *Sterculia Scaphigera* 9 g, and *Periostracum Cicadae* 6 g should be added to clear away heat – evil and benefit the throat.

5. General – Deficiency Type

Main Symptoms and Signs: General deficiency, or infirmity with age, repeated affection of cold; deficiency of qi marked by lassitude, shortness of breath, asthenia, spontaneous perspiration, pale enlarged tongue, and weak floating pulse; deficiency of yang marked by aversion to cold, cold limbs, loose stools, whitish slippery tongue coating, and deep slow pulse; deficiency of blood marked by pale face, lips and nails, dizziness, palpitation, insomnia, pale tongue, and hollow pulse; deficiency of yin marked by dysphoria, feverish sensation in the chest, palms and soles, tidal fever, night sweating, flushed zygomatic region, reddened tongue with little coating, and thready rapid pulse.

Therapeutic Principles: Strengthening the body resistance to relieve exterior syndrome.

Recipe 1. For cold due to deficiency of qi and affection of exopathogenic wind – cold: *Modified Shen su yin (Ginseng and Perilla decoction)*

Radix Ginseng	3 g
Poria	12 g
Herba Schizonepetae	9 g
Folium Perillae	9 g
Radix Peucedani	9 g
Exocarpium Citri Rubrum	9 g
Fructus Aurantii	9 g
Radix Platycodi	9 g
Radix Puerariae	15 g

Radix Aucklandiae 6 g
Pericarpium Citri Reticulatae 6 g
Radix Glycyrrhizae 6 g

Decoct the above ingredients in a right amount of water for oral administration.

Recipe 2. For cold due to deficiency of yang and affection of exopathogenic wind-cold: *Modified zaizao san* (*Rehabilitation powder*).

Radix Aconiti Lateralis Praeparata 6 g
Ramulus Cinnmomi 9 g
Radix Codonopsis 12 g
Radix Astragali 12 g
Radix seu Rhizoma Notopterygii 9 g
Radix Saposhinkoviae 9 g
Rhizoma Ligustici Chuanxiong 9 g
Herba Asari 3 g
Radix Glycyrrhizae 3 g
Rhizoma Zingiberis Recens 3 pcs
Fructus Jujubae 3 dates

Decoct the above ingredients in a right amount of water for oral administration. One dose daily.

Recipe 3. For cold due to deficiency of yin and affection of exopathogenic factors: *Jiajian werrei tang* (*Modified decoction of fragrant Solomonseal*)

Rhizoma Polygonati Odorati 9 g
Radix Cynanchi Atrati 9 g
Herba Menthae 9 g
Radix Platycodi 9 g
Semen Sojae Praeparatum 9 g
Caulis Allii Fistulosi 6 g

Decoct the above ingredients in a right amount of water for oral administration.

Recipe 4. For cold due to deficiency of blood and exopathogenic factors: *Congbai qiwei yin* (*Powder of seven drugs including Chinese green onion stalk*)

Caulis Allii Fistulosi 3 pcs
Radix Puerariae 15 g
Radix Rehmanniae 12 g
Radix Angelicae Sinensis 9 g
Radix Ophiopogonis 9 g
Semen Sojae Praeparatum 9 g

Radix Platycodi 9 g
Rhizoma Zingiberis Recens 3 pcs
Fructus Jujubae 3 dates

Decoct the above ingredients in a right amount of water for oral administration. One dose daily.

COMPLICATIONS

1. **Cold Complicated with Phlegm.** It is manifested by severe cough, sound of the sputum in the throat, or high fever, dyspneic cough with flapping nose, etc.. If it is caused by wind – cold evil, it is proper to dispel the evil from the superficies with drugs of acrid taste and warm nature, release inhibited lung – qi and dissipate phlegm by adding *San'ao tang*. If it is caused by wind – heat, it is appropriate to dispel the evil from the superficies with drugs of acrid and cool nature, remove heat from the lung and dissolve phlegm bu adding *Cortex Mori Radicis* 9 g or using modified *Ma xing shi gan tang* (*Decoction of Ephedra, Apricot kernel, Gypsum and Liquorice*) instead.

If the reveals severe cough, *Ma xing shi gan tang* (*Decoction of Ephedra, Apricot kernel, Gypsum and Liquorice* together with *Semen Lepiddi seu Descurainiae* 6 g and *Ochra Haematitum* 12 g, is applicable to purge the sthenic lung – qi and relieve asthma.

2. **Cold Complicated with Dyspepsia.** It is characterized by poor appetite, fullnes sensation in the chest and abdomen, feverish sensation over the palms and soles, restless night sleep or sour and foul vomiting, stinking stool with indigested food drege, yellowish, thick and greasy fur and strong floating pulse. In this cases, formulae for various kinds of cold can be used by adding *Massa Fermentata* 6 g, *Fructus Hordei Germinatus* 9 g, *Fructus Crataegi* 9 g, *Endothelium Corneum Gigeriae Galli* 3 g, and *Semen Arecae* 9 g to promote digestion. If the fever is not severe but dyspepsia and loose stool may be present, modified *Huoxiang zheng qi san* (*Powder of Agastrachis for restoring health*) is used to expel superficial pathogens and eliminate damp pathogens. The ingredients are: *Folium Perillae* 6 g, *Herba Agastachis* 12 g, *Radix Angelicae Dahuricae* 6 g, *Poria* 9 g, *Rhizoma Atractylodis Macrocephalae* 9 g, *Cortex Magnoliae Officinalis* 9 g, *Rhizoma Pinelliae* 9 g, *Pericarpium Citri Reticulatae* 6 g, *Pericarpium Arecae* 9 g and *Radix Platycodi* 9 g. *Baohe wan* (*Lenitive pill*) may be added, to be taken one pill, three times a day, or *Sixiao pian* is given, 2 – 5 tablets, three times a day.

3. **Cold Complicated with Convulsion.** It is manifested by fever with impeded sweat, flushed face, red eyes, fear and restlessness even convulsion, also called convulsion due to excess of heat. For this case, *Ramulus Uncariae cum Uncis* 6 g, *Bombyx Batry-*

ticatus 9 g, *Periastracum Cicadae* 6 g and *Herba Menthae* 6 g can be added to calm convulsion, stop wind – syndrome and clear away heat. *Niuhuang zhenjing wan* (*Bozoar bolus for stopping convulsion*) or *Hupo baolong wan* can also be added, 0.5 to one pill, twice to three times daily.

OTHER THERAPIES

1. Simple Recipe and Proved Prescription

1) Common cold of wind cold type

(1) Five or six pieces of *Rhizoma Zingiberis Recens*, with some *brown sugar*, are decocted or infused in boiling water for drinking to cause mild perspiration.

(2) Three inches of *Bulbus Allii Fistulosi*, 5 pieces of *Rhizoma Zingiberis Recens* and proper amount of *brown sugar* are decocted for frequent drinking till mild perspiration emerges.

2) Common cold of wind – heat type

(1) *Folium Mori*, *Flos Chrysanthemi*, *Folium Isatidis* or *Radix Isatidis*, all in proper amount, are decocted in water for drinking.

(2) *Fufang Daqingye heji* is given, one injection, 3 times daily.

(3) *Ganmao chongji*, 0.5 to one pack, 3 times daily. The dosage is varied with the ages of young cases.

2. Acupuncture Therapy

1) Wind – cold

Therapeutic Principles: Eliminating wind and relieving the exterior symptoms.

Prescription: Fengmen(BL12), Feishu(BL13), Quchi(LI11), Hegu(LI4).

Supplementary Points: Dazhui(DU14) for fever; Yingxiang(LI20) for nasal obstruction with discharge; Taiyang(EX – HN5) for headache.

Explanation: Fengmen(BL12) and Feishu(BL13) eliminate wind and cold. Quchi (LI11) and Hegu(LI4) relieve the exterior symptoms and clear heat.

2) Wind – heat

Therapeutic Principles: Clearing away heat and relieving the exterior symptoms.

Prescription: Dazhui(DU14), Fengmen(BL12), Feishu(BL13), Quchi(LI11), Hegu(LI4).

Supplementary Points: Yingxiang(LI20) for nasal obstruction with discharge; Yuji (LU10), Shaoshang(LU11) pricked with three – edged needle to cause bleeding for sore throat.

Explanation: Dazhui(DU14), Hegu(LI4) and Quchi(LI11) clear heat and relieve the exterior symptoms. Fengmen(BL12) and Feishu(BL13) promote the lung's function in dispersing and eliminating wind.

3) **Complicated syndromes**

Chize(LU5), Fenglong(ST40) for retention of phlegm;

Zhongwan(RN12), Tianshu(ST25), Qihai(RN6), Zusanli(ST36) for retention of food;

Yintang(EX-HN3), Shenmen(HT7), Yanglingquan(GB34), Taichong(LR3) for convulsion.

Auricular Acupuncture

Prescription: Fei(CO_{14}) lung, Qiguan(CO_{16}) trachea, Neibi(TG_4) internal nose, Erjian($HX_{6,7i}$) ear apex, Wei(CO_4) stomach, Pi(CO_{13}) spleen, Sanjiao(CO_{17}) triple energy.

Method: Two to three points are chosen bilaterally to be needled with strong stimulation. Needles are retained for 10 to 20 minutes.

PREVENTION

1. Attention should be paid to physical training in order to build up health. More out-door activities and sunshine are helpful in resistance against diseases.

2. Clothes should be changed according to different weather, and rooms kept with fresh air.

3. During the epidemic time of the disease, children and cases suffering from cold frequently should not frequently go to public places so as to avoid being infected. When going out, they should wear masks and keep away from those who have got cold.

4. Wash face with cold water, go swimming in winter if possible, in order to strengthen the ability to tolerate cold.

5. Strke a proper balance between work and rest so as to build up the constitution.

6. Take *Yupingfeng san* (*Jade-screen powder*) regularly.

GENERAL NURSING

1. The air in the room should be fresh and well ventilated but the patients should not be in any draught which may worsen the cold. The patients body should be kept warm and the patient's garments and be clothes should be increased according to weather changes.

2. Cases of epidemic influenza should be isolated. The air in the room may be steril-

ized by steaming vinegar, one to two portions of water to one portion of vinegar, and 5－10 ml of vinegar is diluted with water for each cubic meter of room. The sterilization is given once a day or every other day.

3. A mild case does not require rest. But a severe case or one with high fever must rest in bed, getting up only after the fever has subsided, and returning to work only after the symptoms and signs have disappeared. strike a proper balance between work and rest.

4. The patient's food should be nourishing, light and easy to digest, while oily, greasy or sweet food is prohibited. Cases with common cold may eat semifluid food but one with influenza should drink vegetarian fluid diet and plenty of water.

5. Take not of any changes of fever, aversion to cold, sweating, as well as the tongue and pulse condition.

6. Decoction must be decocted for only a short time, not over boiled. One dose of decoction is generally separated into two parts to be taken at different times. But if the symptom of fever improves in a considerable degree and the patient feels much better after taking the first part of the decoction, the other part is prohibited. Sweating, in order to expel pathogenic factors, should not be excessive; mild perspiration over the body is regarded as normal. After sweating, the patient should avoid wind and keep the body warm to avoid any relapse. If the patient does not perspire after taking medicine and the fever continuously rises, a doctor should be informed.

7. The patients should take exercise to build up their disease－resistant ability.

NURSING ACCORDING TO SYNDROME DIFFERENTIATION

1. Wind－cold Syndrome

1) The ward temperature should be a little on the high side.

2) Raw and cold food is prohibited while plenty of hot drinks of water are suitable.

3) Herbs pungent in taste and warm in nature, for relieving the exterior syndrome and venilating the lung and expelling cold should be administered. The selected prescription is *Jing fang baidu san* with modification, the decoction being administered hot. After administration, the patient should be warmly covered and be given more hot water gruel or rice soup to drink in the mean time so as to support the herbal effect.

4) High fever should not be lowered by physiotherapy in order to prevent sweat pores from closing up resulting in retention of pathogenic evils.

5) *Fresh ginger* 3 pieces, *onion* 5 pieces and *prepared soya beans* 9 g are decocted in water for oral use, or *Xiling jiedu pian* taken three times daily.

2. **Wind – heat Syndrome**

1) Keep the ward cool and well ventilated.

2) Plenty of fruits such as water – melon, peach, should be eaten. Drink which is cool in nature such as mung bean soup is suitable.

3) Herbs pungent in flavor and cool in nature should be taken to relieve the exterior syndrome, ventilate the lung and lcear away heat; the prescription is *Yinqiao san* (*Powder of Lonicera and Forsythia*) with modification. The decoction is taken warm, and the patient is kept warm with dry clothes in order to avoid any relapse.

4) *Lophatherum* 12 g, *Herba Menthae* 3 g, *Semen Armeniacae Amarum* 3 g and *Fructus Forsythiae* 3 g are decocted with water for oral use. A sack of *Sangju ganmao chongji* can also be taken orally, three times daily.

3. **Summer – heat Wetness Syndrome**

1) Light and fluid diet is suitable for cases with obvious symptoms of gastrointestinal tract.

2) Herbs are taken to eliminate summer heat from superficies of the body by diaphoresis and eliminate dampness with aromatics. The prescription is *Xinjia xiangru yin* (*Modified decoction of Elsholtzia with supplements*) with modification. The decoction is taken warm. Cases with obvious symptoms of gastrointestinal tract should take the decoction frequently. The amount of each time is small.

3) *Liuyi san* (*Six to one powder*) 12 g and *Herba Menthae* 6 g are taken after being infused in boiling water, or *Huoxiang zhengqi wan* (*Pill of Agastachis for restoring health*) may be taken twice daily.

MASSAGE

Push the forehead outwards for 30 times. Knead Taiyang(EX – HN5) for 30 times. Wipe both the temples outwards for 30 times. Knead Fengchi(GB20) for 30 times. Grasp the posterior cervical ligament for 10 times. Thump Jianjing(GB21) for 20 times. Pat the upper back for 20 times, and pinch and knead Hegu(LI4) for 30 times.

MEDICATED DIET

1. Infuse clean shredded *fresh ginger* 9 g and *brown sugar* 12 g in boiling water. Take the decoction when it is warm. Then the patient is advised to lie in bed with blanket for mild perspiration. It is applicable to wind – cold type.

2. Decoct *chrysanthemum flower* 6 g and *mulberry leaves* 21 g, or infuse them in boiling water. Drink it as tea. It is applicable to wind – heat type.

QIGONG

1. Sit with the legs naturally bent and crossed, with the hands pressing against the ground. Throw out the chest and inhale till the chest is full. Pause for a while; then arch the back and draw in the chest and exhale at the same time. Do for 4 to 5 times. It is applicable to common cold of wind – cold type.

2. Assume the standing or sitting posture. Place both palms flat on their indentical sides of the chest and inhale slowly. During exhalation, read "Si"; meanwhile rub the chest with both palms. Rub for 6 or 12 breaths. It is applicable to comon cold of wind – heat type.

DISCUSSION

It is difficult to evaluate a therapy for the treatment of a self – limited disease like common cold. However, controlled studies have shown that traditional therapy shortened the course of the disease and relieved the symptoms quickly. Traditional therapy has several other advantages. It relieves symptoms without side effects when administered properly. Because the treatment if based on the individual's condition and applied differently to different patients. Chilliness and fever, once relieved, seldom recur, probably because of the anti – virus effect of some ingredients contained in *Radix Ledebouriellae*, *Flos Lonicerae* and *Radix Isatidis*, and because these herbs promote the body's ability to resist disease by regulating yin – yang balance. Research has also shown that *Radix Astragali seu Hedysari*, the main ingredient of *Jade – screen powder*, promotes the blood interferon level induced by virus. This preventive effect, also shown in a double blind controlled test, is of paticular interest in treating individuals vulnerable to recurrent colds.

Chapter Three
Influenza

Influenza, an infectious disease of respiratory tract, is caused by influenza viruses. The idsease has extremely strong infectivity, transmitted by means of droplets. People are very susceptible to influenza and sometimes pandemics may happen over the world. Although influenza may occur at all seasons, it tends to appear during winter and spring. This disease, in traditional Chinese medicine is called *Shixing ganmao*.

MAIN POINTS OF DIAGNOSIS

1. A large number of patients are affected within a short period with clinical features of fever, headache and myalgia.

2. Clinical features

1) The onset of the disease is abrupt, with marked general toxemic symptoms such as chill, fever, headache, myalgia, weakness, etc.

2) Symptoms referable to the respiratory tract such as stuffy nose, rhinorrhea, sore throat and dry cough are usually mild. In some cases, symptoms of the digestive tract such as loss of appetite, nausea, vomiting, abdominal pain and diarrhea may be present.

3) High fever, chest pain, cough, bloody sputum, dyspnea and even coma may occur in severe cases.

4) Physical examination reveals acutely ill complexion and malar flush with congestion of conjunctival and nasopharyngeal mucosa. In patients with influenzal pneumonia or secondary bacterial pneumonia, the respiratory sounds are diminished. Diffuse moist rales may be heard over the lung fields.

3. Laboratory test show a decreased leukocyte count and the ratio of neutrophils to leukocytes, while the lymphocytes count may be relatively elevated. Mucosal imprint from inferior nasal conchae may show inclusions of influenza virus. This is valuable for the early diagnosis. In serological examinations, hemagglutination inhibition test or complement fixation test can be used for the diagnosis. Viral isolation is helpful in confirming the type of pathogen.

DIFFERENTIATION AND TREATMENT OF COMMON SYNDROMES

1. Wind - cold Syndrome

Main Symptoms and Signs: Severe aversion to cold, slight fever, absence of sweat, headache, aching pain of extremities, stuffy nose with nasal discharge, cough with thin sputum, thin and whitish coating of tongue, floating and tight pulse.

Therapeutic Principles: Relieving exterior syndrome with the drugs pungent in flavor and warm in property, ventilating the lung and expelling pathogenic cold.

Recipe: *Modified antiphlogistic powder of Schizonepeta and Ledebouriella*

Herba Schizonepetae	10 g
Radix Ledebouriellae	10 g
Rhizoma seu Radix Notopterygii	10 g
Radix Bupleuri	10 g
Radix Peucedani	10 g
Folium Perillae	10 g
Radix Platycodi	
Rhizoma Zingiberis Recens	3 pcs

Decoct the above ingredients in a right amount of water for oral administration.

Generally, a decoction should be taken in two separate doses a day, one in the morning and the other in the evening. The whole course of treatment covers 3 - 6 successive days, or depends on the patient's condition.

Moreover, supplementary drugs should be added with emphasis on certain symptoms; *Radix Angelicae Dahuricae* 10 g and *Rhizoma Ligustici Chuanxiong* 10 g are used to treat severe headache; *Radix Bupleuri* added to 12 grams and *Herba Menthae* 6 grams for cases with high fever; *Rhizoma seu Radix Notopterygii* 12 grams and 9 grams of *Radix Angelicae Pubescentis* or *Decoction of Notopterygium for rheumatism* is used instead for exhibiting of more symptoms and signs of exterior dampness. If the case is complicated with exterior syndrome of excess characterized by no sweating, headache and pantalgia, severe aversion to cold, *Ephedra decoction* is preferred; If the case is manifested by exterior deficiency with sweating, aversion to wind, slight fever, stuffy nose and retching, *Cinnamon twig decoction* is recommended.

2. Wind - heat Syndrome

Main Symptoms and Signs: High fever, slight aversion to cold, headache, sore throat with congestion, expectoration of yellowish sputum, thirst or even epistaxis, reddened tongue with thin and yellowish fur, floating and rapid pulse.

Therapeutic Principles: Relieving exterior syndrome with the drugs pungent in flavor and cool in property, promoting the dispersing function of the lung and clearing up pathogenic heat.

Recipe: *Modified powder of Lonicera and Forsythia*

Flos Lonicerae	30 g
Fructus Forsythiae	15 g
Radix Isatidis	30 g
Radix Puerariae	20 g
Folium Mori	10 g
Flos Chrysanthemi	10 g
Fructus Arctii	12 g
Herba Lophatheri	10 g
Radix Platycodi	10 g

Decoct the above ingredients in a right amount of water for oral administration.

In addition, the following ingredients should be included with respect to certain symptoms: 30 grams of *Gypsum Fibrosum* for the patients with high fever; 10 grams of *Bulbus Fritillariae Cirrhosae* for patients with severe cough; 10 grams of *Radix Sophorae Subprostratae* and 10 grams of *Radix Scrophulariae* for patients with severe sore throat; 30 grams of *Rhizoma Imperatae* for patients with epistxis; 12 grams of *Radix Bupleuri*, 12 grams of *Radix Scutellariae* and 10 grams of *Rhizoma pinelliae* for patients with alternate spells of fever and chill, nausea and vomiting; 15 grams of *Radix Astragali seu Hedysari* for patients with weak constitution and profuse sweat.

In cases complicated with summer – damp, 10 grams of *Herba Elscholtziae seu Moslae* and 20 grams of *Liuyi san* (*Six to one powder*, wrapped with cloth during decocting) should be administered; In cases of gastro – intestinal influenza pertaining to the syndrome of exterior cold and interior dampness, marked by fever, aversion to cold, vomiting, diarrhea, feeling of fullness and stuffiness in the chest and hypochondrium, thick and greasy fur of the tongue, *Powder of Agastachis for restoring health* is preferred.

Chapter Four

Acute Upper Respiratory Tract Infection

Infection of the respiratory tract is perhaps one of the most common human ailments and is a source of discomfort, disability and loss of time for most average adults. It is also a substantial cause of morbidity and serious illnesses in young children and in the elderly, including inflammation of nasal tract, nasopharynx, pharynx and larynx. Most cases are caused by virus such as *rhinovirus*, *parainfluenza*, *respiratory syncytial virus*, *adenovirus*, *influenza*$_{A, B,}$ and $_{C}$*virus*, etc., but some by bacteria such as *pneumococcus*, *hemolytic streptococcus*, *hemophilus* and *staphylococcus*. Many of these viral infections run their natural course in older children and in adults without specific treatment and without great risk of bacterial complications. In young infants and in the elderly, or in persons with impaired respiratory tract function, bacterial superinfection increases morbidity and mortality rates.

In traditional Chinese medicine, this condition is often called seasonal disease or external affection which refers to the disease or the symptoms caused by the six pathogenic factors, namely *wind*, *cold*, *summer – heat*, *dampness*, *dryness*, *fire*, as well as malignant infection and pathogenic factors. The disease, in traditional Chinese medicine, belongs to the categories of *ganmao* or *shangfeng*, *ru'e*, etc.

Acute upper respiratory tract infections generally are divided into the following five types:

Common cold. This familiar syndrome is characterized mainly by nasal obstruction with discharge, sore throat, sneezing, hoarseness, varying degrees of malaise, cough, sinusitis and otitis. Fever is usually absent in adults but may be present in small children.

Croup (Laryngotracheobronchitis). This is most commonly a parainfluenza virus infection of small children with anatomic location in the subglottal area. It produces hoarseness, a "seal bark" cough and signs of upper airway obstruction with inspiratory stridor xiphoid and suprasternal retraction, but no pain on swallowing.

Herpangina. This disorder is commonly a coxsackie$_{A}$ virus infection of small children with sore throat and fever. The epiglottis is markedly swollen with a cherry red appearance.

Pharyngoconjunctival fever. The causes of this disorder are adenovirus, coxsackie and influenza$_{A, B}$ and $_{C}$virus, and it is characterized mainly by fever, sore throat, increased discharge in the eyes, photophobia and congestion of conjunctiva.

Bacterial pharyngotonsillitis. The most common cause of the illness is hemolytic – streptococcus, pneumococcus and staphylococcus. Its features are abrupt onset with chills and fever, and marked congestion of the pharynx. The temperature is above 39 and the tonsil is enlarged with yellowish exudate on the superficial mucosa.

MAIN POINTS OF DIAGNOSIS

1. Clinical manifestations usually include rhinorrhea, rhinocleisis, sneezing, lacrimation and mild cough. Fever, sore throat, headache, fatigue, poor appetite or vomiting can also be present.

2. Physical examinations may reveal redness of the pharynx with herpes or ulcer in the mouth. Patients with acute tonsillitis may have excessive purulent discharge on the surface of the tonsils and swelling of tonsils. Submaxillary lymphnodes are usually swollen and tender.

3. Laboratory examinations may reveal normal leukocyte count in patients with viral infection, and higher one in those with bacterial infection. X – ray examination of the chest is usually normal.

DIFFERENTIATION AND TREATMENT OF COMMON SYNDROMES

1. Wind – cold Type

Main Symptoms and Signs: Aversion to cold, fever, absence of sweat, stuffy nose, thin nasal discharge, sneezing, mild cough, thin sputum, absence of thirst, headache, itching throat, reddish tongue with thin and white fur, floating and tight pulse, and shallow red superficial venule of the index finger.

Therapeutic Principles: Relieving exterior syndrome with drugs pungent in flavor and warm in property, ventilating the lung and expelling pathogenic cold.

Recipe: *Jingfang baidu san* (*Powder of Schizonepeta and Ledebouriella*)

Herba Schizonepetae 6 g

Radix Ledebouriellae 6 g

Rhizoma seu Radix Notopterygii 9 g

Radix Peucedani 9 g

Radix Platycodi 9 g

Radix Glycyrrhizae 3 g

Decoct the above ingredients in a right amount of water for oral administration.

Besides, in case of headache, 6 grams of *Radix Angelicae Dahuricae* should be added; for those with severe cough, add 6 grams of *Semen Armeniacae* and 9 grams of

Rhizoma Cynanchi Stauntonii.

2. **Wind – heat Type**

Main Symptoms and Signs: Higher fever and milder aversion to cold, headache, stuffy nose, purulent nasal discharge, sneezing, cough with yellowish thick sputum, painful red and swollen throat, dry mouth and thirst, red tongue with thin and white or thin and yellowish fur, floating and rapid pulse, and shallow and clear superficial venule of the index finger with red color.

Therapeutic Principles: Expelling exopathogens from the body surface with drugs of acrid flavour and cool nature, ventilating the lung and clearing away pathogenic heat.

Recipe: *Yinqiao san* (*Modified Powder of Lonicera and Forsythia*)

Flos Lonicerae	9 g
Fructus Forsythiae	9 g
Herba Schizonepetae	6 g
Semen Sojae Praeparatum	6 g
Fructus Arctii	9 g
Herba Menthae	(to be decocted later) 6 g
Herba Lophatheri	6 g
Rhizoma Phragmitis	15 g
Radix Glycyrrhizae	3 g

Decoct the above ingredients in a right amount of water for oral administration.

Besides, in case of high fever, 9 grams of *Radix Bupleuri*, 15 grams of *Radix Puerariae* and 9 grams of *Fructus Gardeniae* should be added. In case of bad headache, 9 grams of *Fructus Viticis* should be added. For those with sore throat, add 9 grams of *Lasiosphaera seu Calvatia*, wrapped in a piece of gauze before it is to be decocted, 9 grams of *Rhizoma Belamcandae* and 12 grams of *Radix Isatidis*. In case of yellow and greasy fur on the tongue, 9 grams of *Semen Coicis* and 12 grams of *Talcum* should be included. For those with severe thirst, 9 grams of *Radix Trichosanthis* should be added. In case of constipation, add 6 grams of *Radix et Rhizoma Rhei* which is to be decocted later, 9 grams of *Radix Scrophulariae* and 9 grams of *Fructus Polygalae Japonica*.

3. **Summer – heat – dampness Type**

Main Symptoms and Signs: High fever, aversion to cold, heaviness sensation in the limbs, fatigue, vomiting, abdominal pain, diarrhea, restlessness, thirst, scanty dark urine, thick and greasy fur on the tongue, and soft and rapid pulse.

Therapeutic Principles: Clearing away summer – heat to relieve the exterior syndrome and removing pathogenic dampness to regulate the stomach.

Recipe: *Xiangru yin* (*Modified Elsholtzia decoction*)

Herba Elscholziae seu Moslae 9 g
Semen Dolichoris Album 15 g
Cortex Magnoliae Officinalis 9 g

Decoct the above ingredients in a right amount of water for oral administration.

Besides, for those with more heat than dampness, omit *Herba Elscholziae seu Moslae*, add 6 grams of *Rhizoma Coptidis*, 12 grams of *Flos Lonicerae*, 12 grams of *Talcum* and 3 grams of *Radix Glycyrrhizae*. In case of more dampness than heat, add 15 grams of *Folium Nelumbinis*, 9 grams of fresh *Herba Elscholziae seu Moslae*, 9 grams of *Herba Eupatorii* and 15 grams of *Exocarpium Citrulli*.

Chapter Five
Acute Bronchitis

Acute bronchitis is an acute inflammation of bronchi. It is a common disease in children, is clinically characterized by cough, expectoration, or dyspnea. In traditional Chinese medicine, it is included in the category of *cough*, *syndrome of dyspnea*, *phlegm retention* and *consumptive lung disease*. Acute bronchitis is an acute inflammation due to infection of bacteria and virus or due to physical or chemical irritation. After it is cured, the affected bronchi may return to normal completely. If the acute inflammation has not been treated timely, it will become protracted and recurrent, which is apt to lead to chronic inflammation of the bronchial mucosa and the peripheral tissues.

ETIOLOGY AND PATHOGENESIS

This disease is caused by both exopathogenic and endopathogenic factors.

1. Exopathogenic Factors

The six exopathogens invade the body and stay in the lung, preventing the lung－qi from flowing freely. Over－intake of liquor and food pungent in flavor and hot in nature or over－smoking will heat the fluid into sputum, blocking the respiratory tract.

2. Endopathogenic Factors

Zang and Fu organs fail to function normally. When the lung is weakened, it can do its duty neither in strengthening *wei qi* so as to keep off exopathogens nor in performing its ascending and descending function. When the spleen is weakened, the fluid will not flow freely, phlegm resulting and staying in the interior. When the kidney is weakened, it will fail to do its duty in receiving air, resulting in dyspnea. The exopathogenic and endopathogenic factors both work to bring about intermittent cough, dyspnea and expectoration, which are protracted and hard to improve.

MAIN POINTS OF DIAGNOSIS

1. Clinical manifestations include fever, unproductive cough, tachypnea, restlessness and poor sleep. Vomiting may occur when cough is severe with discomfort or pain in the chest. After several days, the cough becomes productive and the sputum changes from clear to purulent. There are malaise and loss of appetite in the course of the disease.

2. Results of physical examinations vary with the age of the patients and the stage of the disease. There are signs of nasopharyngitis and conjunctivitis. Auscultation of the chest reveals respiratory harshness, coarse moist rales and high-pitched dry rales.

3. Laboratory examinations show normal or high peripheral blood picture. X-ray examination of the chest is normal or with increased lung-markings.

DIFFERENTIATION AND TREATMENT OF COMMON SYNDROMES

1. Cough due to Pathogenic Wind-cold

Main Symptoms and Signs: Frequent cough with clear and thin sputum, aversion to cold with anhidrosis, fever, headache, stuffy nose with nasal discharge, itching in the throat, hoarseness or general pantalgia with soreness, thin and white fur of the tongue, floating and tight pulse and shallow red superficial venule of the index finger.

Therapeutic Principles: Expelling pathogenic wind-cold and relieving cough by promoting the dispersing function of the lung.

Recipe 1: *San'ao tang (Flavored decoction of three grude drugs)*

Herba Ephedrae	6 g
Semen Armeniacae Amarum	6 g
Radix Glycyrrhizae	3 g
Herba Schizonepetae	6 g
Radix Peucedani	9 g
Rhizoma Pinelliae	6 g
Radix Platycodi	6 g
Bulbus Fritillariae Cirrhosae	9 g

Decoct the above ingredients in a right amount of water for oral administration.

In addition to the above ingredients, 1.5 grams of *Herba Asari* and 9 grams of *Radix Stemonae* are added for those with severe cough. For cases with much sputum, 6 grams of *Exocarpium Citri Reticulatae* should be added.

Recipe 2: *Jiajian huagai san (Modified canopy powder)*

Herba Ephedrae Praeparata	9 g
Semen Armeniacae Amarum	9 g
Exocarpium Citri Rubrum	9 g
Cortex Mori	9 g
Fructus Perillae	9 g
Poria	9 g

Radix Glycyrrhizae 6 g

Decoct the above ingredients in a right amount of water for oral administration. One dose daily.

Modification: When exterior syndrome due to wind – cold is remarkable, the drugs added accordingly are ***Ramulus Cinnamomi*** 9 g, ***Herba Schizonepetae*** 9 g and ***Radix Puerariae*** 12 g. In case of severe cough, ***Bulbus Fritillariae Thunbergii*** 9 g, ***Flos Farfarae*** 12 g, ***Radix Asteris*** 12 g are added. ***Herba Asari*** 3 g, ***Rhizoma Pinelliae*** 9 g and ***Rhizoma Zingiberis*** 9 g added for sneezing, stuffy nose, profuse nasal discharge and plenty of sputum.

Chinese Patent Medicine: *Tongxuan lifei wan* (*Bolus for ventilating and facilitating the flow of lung – qi*). To be taken orally, 6 – 12 g each time, twice daily.

2. **Cough due to Pathogenic Wind – heat**

Main Symptoms and Signs: Cough with unclear throat, yellow and thick sputum which is not easy to be coughed up, sore throat, stuffy nose with turbid nasal discharge, accompanied with fever, headache, slight sweating, red lips and tongue with thin and yellow fur, floating and rapid pulse and shallow purple superficial venule of the index finger.

Therapeutic Principles: Expelling pathogenic wind – heat, relieving cough by promoting the dispersing function of the lung.

Recipe 1: *Sang ju yin* (*Modified decoction of Mulberry leaf and Chrysanthemum*)

Folium Mori 9 g

Flos Chrysanthemi 9 g

Fructus Forsythiae 9 g

Herba Menthae 9 g

Radix Platycodi 9 g

Rhizoma Phragmitis 15 g

Radix Glycyrrhizae 3 g

Semen Armeniacae Amarum 6 g

Decoct the above ingredients in a right amount of water for oral administration.

Besides, in case of severe lung – heat with yellow fur of the tongue, 9 grmas of *Radix Scutellariae* should be added. For those with severe heat in the lung and stomach manifested by strong dyspnea, add 18 grams of *Gypsum Fibrosum*, 9 grams of *Rhizoma Anemarrhenae* and 9 grams of *Semen Lepidii seu Descuraniae*. For those with swollen and sore throat, add 9 grams of *Radix Ophiopogonis*, 9 grams of *Fructus Arctii* and 9 grams of *Rhizoma Bjelamcandae*. In case of much yellow and thick sputum, add 15 grams of *Semen Benincasae*, 6 grams of *Bulbus Fritillariae* and 9 grams of *Fructus Trichosanthis*. 9 grams of *Radix Peucedani* and 9 grams of *Folium Eriobotryae Praepara-*

ta are added for severe cough.

Recipe 2: *Jiawei ma xi shi gan tang* (*Modified decoction of Ephedra, Apricot kernel, Gypsum and liquorice.*)

Flos Lonicerae	30 g
Herba Ephedrae Praeparata	9 g
Bulbus Fritillariae Thunbergii	9 g
Fructus Forsythiae	9 g
Gypsum Fibrosum	30 g
Semen Armeniacae Amarum	9 g
Radix Peucedani	9 g
Radix Glycyrrhizae	3 g

Decoct the above ingredients in a right amount of water for oral administration.

Modification: When there is high fever, flushed face and thirst, the drugs added are *Herba Houttuyniae* 30 g, *Herba Taraxaci* 30 g, *Folium Isatidis* 30 g. In case of reddened and swollen throat, *Lasiophaera seu Calvatia* 9 g, *Fructus Arctii* 9 g and *Bombyx Batryticatus* 9 g are added. When summer-heat is involved, *Herba Nelumbinis* 30 g, *Exocarpium Citrulli* 30 g and *Herba Pogostemonis* 12 g are added.

Chinese Patent Medicine

1: *Zhisou qingguo wan* (*Cough-relieving pill including Chinese white olive*). Taken orally, 9 g each time, twice daily.

2: *Shedan chuanbei ye* (*Mixture of Snake bile and Fritillary bulb*). Taken orally, 10 ml each time, twice daily.

3. Cough due to Pathogenic Wind-dryness

Main Symptoms and Signs: Dry cough without any sputum or with little and mucoid sputum difficult to be coughed up, dry mouth and throat, dry nose, persistent cough with unclear throat, dull pain in both sides of the chest and hypochondrium, constipation, reddened lips and tongue with thin and yellowish or white and dry fur, rapid pulse, and blue and purple superficial venule of the index finger.

Therapeutic Principles: Clearing away lung-heat and moisturizing dryness.

Recipe: *Qingzao jiufei tang* (*Modified decoction for relieving dryness of the lung*)

Gypsum Fibrosum	18 g
Fructus Trichosanthis	12 g
Radix Adenophorae	9 g
Radix Ophiopogonis	9 g
Folium Eriobotryae Praeparata	9 g
Folium Mori	9 g

Semen Armeniacae Amarum 6 g

Rhizoma Anemarrhenae 6 g

Decoct the above ingredients in a right amount of water for oral administration.

For those with continued cough, add 9 grams of *Radix Stemonae* and 9 grams of *Cortex Lycii Radicis*. For those with epistaxis or hemoptysis, add 9 grams of *Radix Rubiae*, 9 grams of *Radix Rehmanniae*, 9 grams of *Scutellariae* and 15 grams of *Rhizoma Imperatae*.

4. Phlegm – heat Gathering in the Lung

Main Symptoms and Signs: Intermittent cough, rapid raucous breathing, rale in the throat due to profuse thick and yellowish sputum, flushed face, fever, bitter taste, thirst, distending pain in the front part of the chest, reddened tongue with yellowish thick coating, and slippery rapid pulse.

Therapeutic Principles: Clearing away heat in the lung to dissolve phlegm, checking upward adverse flow of qi to relieve cough.

Recipe: *Sangbaipi tang* (*Modified decoction of Mulberry bark*) and *Qingjin huatan tang* (*Decoction for removing lung – heat and phlegm*)

Radix Scutellariae 9 g

Rhizoma Coptidis 9 g

Fructus Gardeniae 9 g

Radix Platycodi 9 g

Bulbus Fritillariae Thunbergii 9 g

Exocarpium Citri Rubrum 9 g

Fructus Perillae 9 g

Rhizoma Pinelliae 9 g

Semen Armeniacae Amarum 9 g

Cortex Mori 12 g

Rhizoma Anemarrhenae 12 g

Radix Ophiopogonis 12 g

Fructus Trichosanthis 12 g

Poria 12 g

Decoct the above ingredients in a right amount of water for oral administration.

Modification: When fever is severe, the drugs *Herba Houttuyniae* 30 g, *Herba Patriniae* 30 g and *Rhizoma Paridis* 30 g are added accordingly. In case of severe cough and dyspnea, add *Radix Stemonae* 12 g, *Flos Farfarae* 12 g and *Semen Lepidii seu Descurainiae* 15 g in the recipe. If the patient reveals stuffy nose and yellowish nasal mucus with pus being discharged, *Flos Magnoliae* 12 g, *Semen Benincasae* 30 g and *Semen*

Persicae 9 g are added in the recipe. In case of pain in the chest, the drugs added are *Radix Curcumae* 12 g and *Flos Carthami* 9 g.

5. Dry – heat Impairing the Lung

Main Symptoms and Signs: Uninterrupted cough, dry and itching throat, dry lips and nose, no sputum or little sticky sputum or even with blood, or fever, sligh aversion to cold, headache, stuffy nose, reddened tongue tip, thin yellowish and dry tongue coating, and floating and a bit rapid pulse.

Therapeutic Principles: Dispelling wind and clearing away heat, moistening the lung and arresting cough.

Recipe: *Sang xing tang* (*Decoction of Mulberry leaf and Apricot kernel*)

Folium Mori	9 g
Semen Armeniacae Amarum	9 g
Bulbus Fritillariae Thunbergii	9 g
Semen Sojae Praeparatum	9 g
Fructus Gardeniae	9 g
Radix glehniae	12 g
Exocarpium Pyrus	15 g

Decoct the above ingredients in a right amount of water for oral administration.

Modification: If the body fluid has been impaired more severely, *Radix Ophiopogonis* 15 g and *Herba Dendrobii* 30 g are suitable to be added. In case of blood – stained sputum and epistaxis, *Rhizoma Imperatae* 30 g, *Nodus Nelumbinis Rhizomatis* 30 g, *Rhizoma Anemarrhenae* are added.

Chapter Six
Chronic Bronchitis

Chronic bronchitis causes increased mucous secretion in the tracheobronchial tract, resulting in a productive cough which is present on most days for a minimum of three months of the year and for at least two consecutive years. It is the most common debilitating respiratory disease in China as well as in other countries, particularly among the aged.

Its cause is not yet clear, but several factors are strongly associated with this disease. **Cigarette smoking** has been shown to be the most important predisposing factor. Some doctors hold that *pneumococci* and *hemophilus* cause infections that result in chronic bronchitis. However, others believe that the infections are the result rather than the cause of this chronic disease. Endogenous factors may also be involved. A genetic abnormality that affects mucus production may impair bronchial clearance and harm protective mechanisms, leading to recurrent or chronic infection. Bronchial allergies may increase secretion of mucus or cause one to be more susceptible to bronchial infection. Exposure to cold exacerbates the condition and may also be related to constitutional hypersensitivity.

Goblet cells in the epithelial lining and bronchial mucous glands lying beneath the epithelium produce the secretion of the tracheobronchial trees. In chronic bronchitis, the mucous glands increase in thickness, and goblet cells increase in number. These changes, along with an increase in the volume of tracheobronchial secretions, explain the chronic productive cough. But late in the course of chronic bronchitis, severe airway obstruction usually occurs, and this cannot be entirely explained by the narrowing of central airways caused by mucous gland thickening and obstruction by the secretions themselves. Small airway obstruction resulting from goblet cell proliferation or bronchiolitis may play an important role. Other morphologic changes accompanying goblet cell and bronchial gland abnormalities include fragmentation of the mucosa, destruction of cilia, inflammatory cell infiltration of the epithelium and subepithelium and basal cell hyperplasia and squamous metaplasia of columnar epithelium. Once ciliated mucosae have been disrupted, airway defense becomes more susceptible to subsequent injury.

Owing to the complexity of its pathogenesis and pathological changes, chronic bronchitis is difficult to treat, especially where a long-term cure is concerned.

In traditional Chinese medicine, chronic bronchitis is closely linked to *cough*, *phlegm* and *dyspnea* in syndrome diagnosis and treatment.

ETIOLOGY AND PATHOGENESIS

The hallmarks of chronic bronchitis are a chronic cough and sputum production. Shortness of breath may later become prominent. From the traditional point of view, cough is a common symptom of lung disease, but the production of sputum is not necessarily confined to disorders of the lungs. Purulent sputum usually results when exogenous pathogenic factors, particularly heat, attack the lungs. Production of nonpurulent voluminous phlegm is often attributed to dysfunction of the spleen. In this case, the lungs merely store the phlegm and cough it up. Accumulation of phlegm in the lungs renders them vulnerable to repeated attacks by exogenous pathogenic factors, resulting in acute exacerbations. Shortness of breath with difficulty in exhalation, usually occurring late in the course of chronic bronchitis indicates that the kidneys are involved, since they help the lungs respire, and protracted difficulty in respiration with prolonged exhalation is characteristic of impaired kidneys.

In summary, traditional Chinese medicine considers chronic bronchitis a disease of the lungs that also involves impairment of the functions of the spleen and the kidneys. Only during acute exacerbations do exogenous pathogens play an important role.

MAIN POINTS OF DIAGNOSIS

1. Productive cough is present on most days for a minimum of 3 months in the year (in at least two consecutive years).

2. During relatively quiescent period, the only finding may be increased anteroposterior diameter of the chest. Other findings such as hyperresonance to percussion, prolonged expiratory phase, scattered diffuse coarse or moderate rhonchi and rale and wheezing are also present.

3. Chest x-ray shows evidence of pulmonary overinflation with increased anteroposterior diameter, flattened diaphragm and increased retrosternal air space. There often prominent and increased bronchial markings at the lung base as parallel or tapering shadows (*tram lines*) which reflect the increased thickness of the bronchial wall.

DIFFERENTIATION AND TREATMENT OF COMMONSYNDROMES

The patient should be vigorously encouraged to discontinue cigarette smoking and avoid exposure to other toxic inhalants and postural drainage exercises when possible. In traditional Chinese medicine, the general rule of herbal treatment for chronic bronchitis is to relieve cough, to invigorate or reinforce the function of the lungs, spleen and/or kidneys. However, if acute exacerbation exists, priority should be given to removing the pathogenic factors.

1. Wind – cold Cough

Main Symptoms and Signs: Cough, thin and white sputum, itching of the throat, accompanied by aversion to cold, fever, anidrosis, nasal obstruction and discharge. Thin and white tongue coating, superficial pulse.

Therapeutic Principles: Promote the dispersing function of the lung and dispel cold to relieve cough.

Recipe:

leaf of purple perilla	9g
fresh ginger	3 pieces
peucedanum root	9 g
apricot kernel	9 g
platycodon root	9 g
licorice root	6 g

Patent Medicine: *Lung – ventilating – regulating bolus* (*Tongxuan lifei wan*). Take 2 boluses each time, 3 times a day.

2. Wind – heat Cough

Main Symptoms and Signs: Cough with yellow and thick sputum, or dry cough, thirst and sore throat, accompanied by fever, aversion to wind, sweating. Thin and yellow tongue coating, superficial and rapid pulse.

Therapeutic Principles: Dispel wind and remove heat, eliminate phlegm and relieve cough.

Recipe:

mulberry leaf	9 g
bitter apricot kernel	9g
platycodon root	9 g
reed rhizome	9 g

chrysanthemum flower	6 g
pepermint	6 g
licorice root	6 g
forsythia fruit	15 g

Patent Medicine: *Fufang shendan chuanbei san* (*Compound powder of Snake - bile and Fritillary bulb*). Take 0.6 g each time, 3 times a day (for young children 0.3 g each time).

3. **Phlegm - damp Attacking the Lung**

Main Symptoms and Signs: Cough with profuse white and sticky sputum, stuffiness and oppression of the chest, loss of appetite. White and greasy tongue fur, slippery pulse.

Therapeutic Principles: Invigorate the spleen and dry the dampness, reduce phlegm and relieve cough.

Recipe:

tangerine peel	15 g
pinellia tuber	15 g
poria	15 g
atractylodes rhizome	9 g
magnolia bark	9 g
aster root	9 g
coltsfoot flower	9 g
licorice root	6 g

Patent Medicine: *Tankejing pian* (*Expectorant tablets*). Take one tablet in the mouth each time, 3 times a day.

4. **Deficiency of the Lung - yin**

Main Symptoms and Signs: Dry mouth without sputum or with scanty sputum, dryness of the nose and throat, sore throat, expectoration with blood or hemoptysis, hectic fever, malar flush. Red tongue with scanty coating, thready and rapid pulse.

Therapeutic Principles: Nourish yin and clear away the lung - heat, remove phlegm and relieve cough.

Recipe:

glehnia root	30 g
ophiopogon root	9 g
fragrant solomonsealrhizome	9 g
trichosanthes root	9 g
hyacinth bean	9 g
fritillary bulb	9 g

apricot kernel	9 g
stellaria root	6 g
wolfberry bark	6 g
scutellaria root	6 g
licorice root	6 g

Patent Medicine: *Run fei gao* (*Lung – nourishing semifluid extract*). Take 15 g each time, 3 time a day.

5. Deficiency of the Spleen

Main Symptoms and Signs: Profuse production of phlegm. In addition to the respiratory symptoms, patients often complain of loss of appetite, abdominal distension and loose stools. The coating is often whitish and greasy, and the pulse is slippery.

Therapeutic Principles: Tonify the spleen and eliminate phlegm.

Recipe: *Er chen tang* (*Decoction of two old drugs*)

Rhizoma Pinellia	15 g
Pericarpium Citri Reticulatae	15 g
Poria	9 g
Radix Glycyrrhizae Praeparata	3 g

Add 3 grams of *ginger* and a piece of *black plum* into the above recipe, and then decoct them in water for oral use.

6 Deficiency of the Kidneys

Main Symptoms and Signs: Shortness of breath with prolonged expiration accompanied by coughing and expectoration. The patient may feel an aversion to cold with cold extremities, soreness in the loins, limpness in the legs and nocturia. The pulse is thready and weak, especially at the cubit.

Therapeutic Principles: Tonify the kidneys and relieve dyspnea.

Recipe: *Duqi wan* (*Dyspnea – relieving pill*), composed of *Liuwei dihuang wan* (*Bolus of six ingredients including Rehmannia*), a common formula for tonifying the kidney, and *Fructus Schisandrae*, an ingredient for relieving cough and dypnea. If marked cold symptoms are present, such as aversion to cold and cold extremities, *Radix Aconiti Praeparata* and *Cortex Cinnamomi* are added.

7. Acute Exacerbation of the Cold Type

Main Symptoms and Signs: Usually precipitated by catching a cold and manifested by an aggravated cough and expectoration of voluminous thin sputum, whitish in color. The pulse is often floating and tense.

Therapeutic Principles: Dispel cold, warm the lungs, arrest cough and relieve asthma.

Recipe: *Xiaoqinglong tang* (*Minor decoction of Blue dragon*)

Herba Ephedrae (with joins removed)	9 g
Radix Paeoniae	9 g
Herba Asari	3 g
Rhizoma Zingiberis	3 g
Radix Glycyrrhizae Praeparata	6 g
Ramulus Cinnamomi	6 g
Rhizoma Pinelliae	9 g
Fructus Schisandrae	3 g

Decoct the above ingredients in a right amount of water for oral administration.

In this formula, ***Herba Ephedrae***, ***Ramulus Cinnamomi***, ***Herba Asari*** and ***Rhizoma Zingiberis*** combine to expel cold, mostly through diaphoresis. Modern research has shown, however, that ***Herba Ephedrae*** not only causes diaphoresis but also has bronchodilatory, anti-inflammatory, anti-allergic, anti-pyretic and anti-viral actions. Apparently, these actions help control an actue exacerbation, whether it was caused by an upper respiratory viral infection or by an allergic mechanism related to exposure to cold or allergens. *Radix Cinnamomi* can cause dilatation of the peripheral blood vessels and has antibacterial (e.g., anti-pneumococcic) and anti-viral (e.g., anti-influenzal) actions. *Rhizoma Zingiberis* is also a vasodilator. ***Herba Asari*** is both an antipyretic and an analgesic.

Rhizoma Pinelliae Praeparata is another important ingredient in this formula. It is a phlegm-resolving drug indicated for treating excessive thin sputum but not for purulent viscid sputum. Modern research has shown that it can inhibit the secretion induced by pilocarpine. Therefore, it is not an expectorant in modern medicine.

8. Acute Exacerbation of the Heat Type

Main Symptoms and Signs: Purulent sputum and may be accompanied by fever, dryness of the mouth, concentrated urine and constipation. The tongue coating is usually yellow, the pulse rapid and slippery.

Therapeutic Principles: Clear the pathogenic heat in the lungs, eliminate phlegm and relieve cough.

Recipe: *Qingjin huatan tang* (*Decoction for clearing the lungs and resolving phlegm*)

Radix Scutellariae	9 g
Fructus Gardeniae	9 g
Radix Ophiopogonis	9 g
Rhizoma Anemarrhenae	9 g
Radix Platycodi	9 g
Cortex Mori Radicis	9 g

Bulbus Fritillariae Thunbergii	9 g
Semen Trichosanthis	9 g
Exocarpium Citri Granis	9 g
Poria	9 g
Radix Glycyrrhizae	3 g

Compared with *Xiaoqinglong tang*, this formula has more ingredients with broad antibacterial actions, such as *Radix Scutellariae*, *Fructus Gardeniae*, *Radix Ophiopogonis* and *Rhizoma Anemarrhenae*, and more potent antipyretic ingredients, such as *Radix Scutellariae*, *Radix Platycodi* and *Rhizoma Anemarrhenae*. The phlegm – resolving ingredients contained in this formula, such as *Radix Platycodi* and *Bulbus Fritillariae Cirrhosae* also differ from *Rhizoma Pinelliae Praeparata*. They are expectorants that increase and liquefy bronchial secretions, thus making the phlegm easier for the patient to cough up and spit out.

ACUPUNCTURE AND MOXIBUSTION

1. Body Acupuncture

Main Points: Feishu(BL13).

Complementary Points: Add Lieque(LU7) and Hegu(LI4) for wind – cold cough; Dazhui(DU14) and Waiguan(SJ5) for wind – heat cough; Fenglong(ST40), Zhongwan (RN12), Chize(LU5) and Zusanli(ST36) for phlegm – damp attacking the lung; Zhongfu(LU1), Zhaohai(KI6) and Lieque(LU7) for insufficiency of the lung yin.

Method: Use filiform needles to puncture the points with reducing method during the seizure period and reinforcing method or even manipulation during the remission period.

2. Auricular Acupuncture

Prescribed Points: Qiguan(CO_{16}), Fei(CO_{14}), Shenmen(TF_4), Zhen(AT_3).

Method: Give a moderate or strong stimulation. Retain the needles for 30 minutes. The seed – embedding method may also be used. two or three points are selected for each treatment.

MASSAGE

For the wind – cold and wind – heat typee, push Cuanzhu(BL2) and Kangong; knead Taiyang(EX – HN5); clear the Lung Meridian; move Neibagua: push and knead Danzhong(RN17); knead Rupang(EX – CA) and Rugen(ST18); knead Feishu(BL130; push the scapulae respectively.

For phlegm – damp attacking the lung and insufficiency of the lung – yin, reinforce the Lung Meridian and Spleen Meridian; push Neibagua; push and knead Danzhong (RN17); knead Rupang(EX – CA) and Ruen(ST18); knead Zhongwan(RN12) and Feishu(BL13); press and knead Zusanli(ST36).

MEDICATED DIET

1. Steam 30 g of *honey*, one piece of *white radish*, 3 g of *dried ginger* and 3 g of *ephedra* together in a bowl; when they are done, take out *ginger* and *ephedra*, and eat the *honey* and *radish*. It is suitable to the wind – cold type.

2. Infuse *chrysanthemum flower* 9 g, *bitter apricot kernel* 6 g, *mulberry leaf* 6 g and *licorice root* 3 g in boiling water to drink as tea. It is suitable to the wind – heat type.

3. Decoct 12 g of *red tangerine peel* and 6 g of *apricot kernel* in water first and sift the liquid from the dregs. Then add *polished rounded – grained rice* 50 g and a right amount of water into the liquid to make gruel. Take the gruel once or twice a day. It is suitable to the type of phlegm – damp attacking the lung.

4. Cut 250 g of *water chestnut*, 250 g of *fresh lotus root*, 250 g of*white radish* and 500 g of *pear* into pieces and extract their juice; then add 250 g of honey in it and mix them well; keep the honeyed juice in a refrigerater. Take the juice twice to three times a day, , 30 ml each time. It is used for the type of insufficiency of the lung yin.

QIGONG

1. Assume the sitting or standing posture. Gently place the right palm flat on the location of Zhongwan(RN12) on the upper abdomen and exhale slowly. When exhaling, rub it with the right palm clockwise. Meanwhile, read “hu”. Do for 10 or 20 breaths.

2. Assume the standing posture. Naturally relax the whole body, breathe naturally, take the waist as an axis and bring both arms to swing to the left and right. Look rightward when swinging to the left and look leftward when swinging to the right, with the mind focusing on the heels. Then assume the kneeling posture, puts the palms levelly on a bed and pause for a while. Turn the head leftward and backward and look into the distance with the eyes wide open. Then turn the head rightward and backward and look with the eyes wide open. Do for 5 times in the left and right respectively.

The above two methods are good for the exterior syndrome.

3. Relax the whole body. Breathe naturally and get rid of the distracting thoughts.

First knock the teeth for 36 times. Stir saliva inside the mouth with the tongue and swallow the saliva in three parts. Send it with the mind to the middle chest and lower Dantian. Then imagine a white qi; when inhaling, fill the whole mouth with it; when exhaling, send the qi slowly to the lungs and down to Dantian and further into the skin and hair of the whole body. Do for 9 or 18 times. It is good for insufficiency of the lung – qi and lung – yin.

4. Sit with the legs naturally bent and crossed. Place the palms on the knees. First turn leftwards for 4 times and then turn rightwards for 4 times. Inhale when turning leftwards and bend forwards to exhale. Finally assume the standing or sitting posture. Place both palms flat on their identical sides of the chest and inhale slowly. When exhaling, read "Si". In the mean time, rub the chestt with both palms. Rub for 6 or 12 breaths. The method is good for the type of phlegm – damp attacking the lung.

NEW EFFECTIVE HERBAL DRUGS

In recent decades, researchers have tested hundreds of species of herbs for their effects in treating chrronic bronchitis. Since the criteria for assessing effectiveness in most studies were based on the control of cough, expectoration and asthma, these new herbs are useful mainly for symptomatic relief.

Oleum Cymopogonis, is a bronchodilator effective for chronic bronchitis and bronchial asthma. It is available in an aerosol spray for inhalation.

Oleum Rhododendri Daurici, is both an antitussive and an expectorant. It is available in capsules for oral administration. The usual dose for chronic bronchitis is 0.05 – 0.1 grams, two to three times daily.

Oleum Viticis Negundo, is an expectorant, antitussive and antiasthmatic. It is available in capsules for oral administration. The usual dose for chronic bronchitis is 20 – 40 mg, 3 times daily.

Oleum Artemisiae Lactiflorae, is also an expectorant and antiasthmatic, slightly more potent than *Oleum Viticis Negundo*. Its usual dose is 20 mg, 3 times a day.

MODERN APPLICATION OF TRADITIONAL PRESCRIPTIONS

Since chronic bronchitis results from impaired functioning of the lungs, spleen and kidneys, it is rational to seek better combinations of tonics to strengthen these organs. Specialists have developed various formulae for this purpose, most of which are modifications of traditional ones. Many have proven effective in clinical sutdies, and some of them have been generally accepted.

Tanyin wan (*Pill for treating fluid – phlegm*). It is composed of *Rhizoma Atractylodis*, *Rhizoma Atractylodis Macrocephalae*, *Rhizoma Zingiberis*, *Radix Aconiti Lateralis Praeparata*, *Cortex Cinnamomi*, *Radix Glycyrrhizae*, *Semen Sinapis*, *Fructus Perillae* and *Semen Raphani*. This formula combines two traditional prescriptions: *Fugui lizhong tang* (*Decoction for regulating the spleen function with Cinnamon and Aconite*) and *Sanzi tang* (*Decoction of three kinds of seeds*). The former is a traditional formula ofr invigorating the spleen with *Radix Aconiti Lateralis Praeparata* and *Cortex Cinnamomi* for invigorating the function of the kidneys; the latter is a traditional formula ofr symptomatic relief of cough and expectoration.

Among the three organs involved in chronic bronchitis, the kidneys seem to be the most important, usually beomces more and more pronounced as the disease develops. Researchers began to ask whether invigorating the kidney function should be the chief apporach to treating chronic bronchitis. A group of 522 cases with chronic bronchitis was treated. Of these patients, 64 received only antibiotics and expectorants during acute exacerbations. They were the control group. The remaining 458 patients received the same treatment during acute exacerbation, but in addition received *Kidney tonic tablets* from September to April each year to prevent the acute exaceerbations that typically occur in winter. Doctors chose patients in the control group and the kidney tonic groups at random, but obserbved only two control groups and the kidney tonic groups made subsequent control groups unnecessary. Of the 34 cases treated with *Kidney tonic tablets* from 1973 to 1975, 62.5 percent showed marked improvement (as shown in a five – year follow – up study) and 28.1 percent experienced a clinical cure. These results confirmed the importance of invigorating the kidney function in the treatment of chronic bronchitis.

Researchers used two kinds of *Kidney tonic tablets* in these studies. *Wen yang pian* (*Kidney tonic tablet for yang deficiency*, which is composed of *Radix Rehmanniae*, *Rhizoma Dioscoroeae*, *Herba Epimedii*, *Fructus Psoraleae*, *Semen Cuscutae* and *Pericarpium Citri reticulatae*, is indicated for chronic bronchitis. It in the course of treatment with *Wen yang pian* thirst and constipation occur, indicating the presence of heat manifestation, *Zi yin pian* (*Kidney tonic tablet for yin deficiency* should be added. It contains *Radix Rehmanniae*, *Radix Asparagi*, *Rhizoma Dioscoreae*, *Rhizoma Polygonati*, *Fructus Ligustri Lucid* and *Pericarpium Citri Reticulatae*.

In another report researchers used *Guben wan* (*Pill for strengthening the constipation*) to treat chronic bronchitis with satisfactory results. This pill is composed of *Radix Astragali*, *Rhizoma Atractylosdis Macrocephalae*, *Radix Ledebouriellae*, *Radix Codonopsis Pilosulae*, *Poria*, *Radix Glycyrrhizae*, *Pericarpium Citri Reticulatae*, *Rhizoma*

Pinelliae, *Fructus Psoraleae* and *Placenta Hominis*.

Kidney tonic tablets chiefly contain kidney tonics, whereas *Guben wan* contains spleen tonics. However, the effect of the latter was comparable to that of the former. In a long–term treatment of 140 chronic bronchitics for three–to–five years, 23 (16.4 percent) were clinically cured, 76 (54.3 percent) showed marked improvement and 26 (18.6 percent) improved, the total effective rate being 89.3 percent. In a control group in which physicians gave the patients only smptomatic treatment during acute exacerbation, 4.2 percent showed marked improvement and 33.3 percent improved, for a total effective rate of 37.5 percent.

It is interesting to note that in experimental studies both *Kidney tonic tablets* and *Guben wan*, as well as *Tanyin wan*, stimulate the pituitary–adrenal system and enhance the immune functions of the body. These actions may be the reason for the effect of these toncis on chronic bronchitis.

Chapter Seven
Bronchiectasis

Bronchiectasis is included in the category of *cough*, *phlegm*, *lung abscess* and *hemoptysis* in traditional Chinese medicine. Its main symptoms are chronic cough, profuse pyoid sputum and intermittent hemoptysis.

Bronchiectasis means dilatation and deformation of the bronchi due to damage of the bronchus walls caused by inflammation of the bronchi and their peripheral tissues. Usually, it is followed by infection of the bronchi and lung, and is commonly seen in children and young people.

ETIOLOGY AND PATHOGENESIS

Weakned constitution, repeated catching of cold, prolonged cough and pulmonary tuberculosis lead to deficiency of vital energy, which tends to provide the change for exopathogens to attack. Dysfunction of the **Zang-fu** organs leads to formation of phlegm in the interior, providing endopathogen. Exopathogen and endopathogen get together to result in protracted cough and expectoration. The disease is thus developed. In a part of the patients, it is caused by the affection of noxious-heat, or by the attack of cold-pathogen prolonged retention of which brings about stasis of blood, accumulation of phlegm and even damage of the lung vessels. In this case, it is manifested by pyoid sputum and hemoptysis. If the noxious-heat is excessive and lingering, **qi** will be exhausted and **yin** damaged, which is, in turn, marked by syndrome of deficiency complicated by excess.

DIFFERENTIATION AND TREATMENT OF COMMON SYNDROMES

1. Type of Phlegm Obstructing the Lung

Main Symptoms and Signs: Protracted cough, spitting out after getting up in the morning or going to bed at night profuse sputum which may be divided into three layers after standing still for several hours, distention and fullness in the chest and even nausea and vomiting when there is difficulty in expectoration, the cough and asthma relieved after the sputum has been spitted up, white greasy tongue coating, and taut slippery pulse.

Therapeutic Principles: Eliminate dampness and phlegm, regulate the flow of qi to relieve depression in the chest.

Recipe: *Jiajian daotan tang* (*Decoction for expelling phlegm*)

Pericarpium Citri Reticulatae	9 g
Rhizoma Pinelliae	9 g
Poria	12 g
Fructus Aurantii Immaturus	9 g
Arisaema cum Bile	9 g
Radix Glycyrrhizae	6 g

Decoct the above ingredients in a right amount of water for oral administration.

Modification: If there is severe cough, the drugs added are: *Semen Armeniacae Amarum* 9 g, *Bulbus Fritillariae Thunbergii* 9 g and *Cortex Magnoliae Officinalis* 9 g.

Add *Caulis Bambusae in Taeniam* 12 g for nausea and vomiting.

Rhizoma Zingiberis 9 g, *Herba Asari* 3 g and *Semen Sinapis Alba* 9 g added for cold - natured symptoms.

Succus Bambosae 20 - 30 ml and *Semen Trichosanthis* 24 g added for difficulty in expectoration.

Chinese Patent Medicine 1: *Juhong wan* (*Red tangerine peel pill*). Taken orally, 12 g each time, twice daily.

Chinese Patent Medicine 2: *Fufang jiegeng pian* (*Composite tablet of Platycodon root*). Taken orllay, 3 - 4 tablets each time, 3 times daily.

2. Type of Retention of Noxious - heat and Phlegm

Main Symptoms and Signs: Profuse yelowish - green sputum sometimes with foul odour, high fever, oppressed sensation in the chest, rapid breathing, reddened tongue with yellow greasy coating, and slippery rapid forceful pulse.

Therapeutic Principles: Clear away heat in the lung, detoxicate and remove retained phlegm.

Recipe: *Jiajian huanglian jiedu tang* (*Modified antidotal decoction of Coptis*), *Qianjin weijing tang* (*Reed stem decoction*) and *Jiegeng tang* (*Decoction of Platycodon*)

Rhizoma Coptidis	9 g
Radix Scutellariae	9 g
Cortex Phellodendri	6 g
Fructus Gardeniae	9 g
Rhizoma Phragmitis	30 g
Semen Persicae	9 g
Semen Coicis	30 g
Semen Benincasae	30 g

Radix Platycodi 15 g

Radix Glycyrrhizae 6 g

Decoct the above ingredients in a right amount of water for oral administration.

Modification: In case of cough and dyspnea which make the patient only sit with the back supported rather than lie down, *Semen Armeniacae Amarum* 9 g, *Semen Lepidii seu Descurainiae* 24 g and *Cortex Mori* 24 g are added.

In case of high fever, *Herba Houttuyniae* 30 g, *Flos Lonicerae* 30 g and *Flos Chrysanthemi Indici* 30 g are added.

In case of constipation, *Radix et Rhizoma Rhei* 9 g and *Natrii Sulfas* 9 g are added.

3. Lung – vessels Injured by Heat

Main Symptoms and Signs: Sputum with blood, even repeated spitting of bright red blood in large quantity, reddened tongue with yellow coating, and deep rapid pulse.

Therapeutic Principles: Clear away lung – heat, cooling blood and stopping bleeding.

Recipe: *Jiajian xijiao dihuang tang* (*Modified decoction of Rhinoceros horn and Rehmannia*)

Cornu Rhinocerotis (taken after being infused in water) 1.5 g

Radix Rehmanniae 30 g

Cortex Moutan 9 g

Radix Paeoniae Alba 9 g

Rhizoma Imperatae 30 g

Nodus Nelumbinis Rhizomatis 30 g

Decoct the above ingredients in a right amount of water for oral administration.

Modification: In case of blood spitted out in large quantity, the drugs considerably added are *Herba Agrimoniae* 30 g, *Cacumen Platycodi* 30 g and *Rhizoma Bletillae* (in the form of powder and taken after being infused in water) 9 g.

In case of sputum with pus, *Rhizoma Fagopyri Cymosi* 30 g, *Fructus Forsythiae* 15 g, *Herba Patriniae* 30 g, *Radix Platycodi* 9 g and *Semen Coicis* 30 g are added.

Chinese Patent Medicine: *Daige san* (*Powder of natural Indigo and Clam shell*). Taken orally, 1.5 – 3 g each time, 1 – 2 times daily.

4. Yin – impairment and Qi – exhaustion

Main Symptoms and Signs: Protracted cough often with pyoid or bloody sputum, emaciation, lassitude, tidal fever in the afternoon, feverish sensation in the palms and soles, enlarged tender tongue with exfoliative fur, and thready rapid weak pulse.

Therapeutic Principles: Invigorate qi and nourish yin, clear away lung – heat and eliminate phlegm.

Recipe: *Jiajian shengmai san* (*Pulse – activating powder*), *Yangyin qingfeitang* (*Decoction for nourishing yin and clearing lung – heat*)

Radix Ginseng	3 g
Radix Ophiopogonis	15 g
Fructus Schisandrae	6 g
Radix Rehmanniae	15 g
Radix Scrophulariae	15 g
Bulbus Fritillariae Thunbergii	9 g
Cortex Moutan	12 g

Decoct the above ingredients in a right amount of water for oral administration.

Modification: For tidal fever, *Cortex Lycii* 30 g, *Radix Cynanchi Atrati* 9 g and *Rhizoma Anemarrhenae* 12 g are added.

For hemoptysis, *Herba Ecliptae* 9 g, *Herba Cirsii* 30 g, and *Radix Rubiae* are added.

For cough, *Semen Armeniacae Amarum* 9 g, *Radix Stemonae* 12 g, and *Bulbus Lilii* 30 g are added.

For pyoid sputum, *Herba Taraxaci* 30 g and *Herba Violae* 30 g are added.

For severe deficiency of qi, *Radix Astragali* 24 g is added.

5. Injury of the Lung by Wind – heat

Main Symptoms and Signs: Tickling sensation in the throat, cough, sputum with blood, dry mouth and nose, or accompanied by fever. Red tongue with thin and yellow coating, superficial and rapid pulse.

Therapeutic Principles: Clear away heat and moisten the lung.

Recipe:

mulberry leaf	9 g
apricot kernel	9 g
glehina root	15 g
pear peel	9 g
capejasmine fruit	9 g
honeysuckle flower	12 g
forsythia fruit	12 g
cogongrass rhizome	15 g
lotus node	12 g

6. Invasion of the Liver – fire into the Lung

Main Symptoms and Signs: Paroxysmal cough, sputum with blood streak, or with fresh red blood, dragging pain in the chest and hypochondrium during cough, irritability, temperament, constipated stools, scanty and brown urine. Red tongue with thin and yellow coating, wiry and rapid pulse.

Therapeutic Principles: Clean the liver and clear away the lung heat.

Recipe:

mulberry bark	12 g
wolfberry bark	9 g
clam shell	12 g
natural indigo	6 g
moutan bark	9 g
scutellaria root	12 g
capejasmine fruit	12 g
fresh rehmannia root	12 g
eclipta	12 g
hairyvein agrimony	30 g

4. **Accumulation of Phlegm – heat in the Lung**

Main Symptoms and Signs: Cough, chest pain, yellow and thick sputum or with bloody thread, coarse breathing, thirst, yellow and brown urine. Dry tongue with yellow coating, surging and large pulse or slippery and rapid pulse.

Therapeutic Principles: Clear away heat and dissolve toxicity, promote the dispersing function of the lung and dissipate phlegm.

Recipe:

ephedra	9 g
apricot kernel	9 g
gypsum	30 g
reed rhizome	30 g
waxgourd seed	12 g
peach kernel	9 g
coix seed	15 g
tabasheer	9 g
dayflower	60 g
licorice	6 g

SIMPLE AND CONVENIENT RECIPE

1. Smash fresh *hairy vein agrimony* 250 g to ge fjuice. Add *lotus juice* 50 ml. Steam it warm and then take it after it becomes cool.

2. Decoct *imperata rhizome* 30 g. Take it after it is infused with 100 ml *baby's urine*.

ACUPUNCTURE AND MOXIBUSTION

1. Body Acupuncture

Main Points: Feishu(BL13), Zhongfu(LU1), Chize(LU5), Fenglong(ST40), Kongzui(LU6), and Hegu(LI4).

Complementary Points: Add Dazhui(DU14) and Taixi(KI3) for fever; add Yinxi (HT6) and Fuliu(KI7) for night sweating.

Method: The filiform needles are punctured with sedation and retained for 30 minutes. The treatment is given once every day, and 10 days of treatment consisted of one course.

2. Auricular Acupuncture

Prescribed Points: Fei(CO_{14}) lung, Qiguan(CO_{16}) trachea.

Method: The filiform needles are punctured with strongstimulation and retained for 20 minutes. The bleeding method can be applied on the ear apex in addition in severe hemoptysis.

MASSAGE

Chafe Dazhui(DU14) for 20 times. Press and knead Feishu(BL13) and Pishu (BL20) for 20 times respectively. Rub Zhongwan(RN12) for 30 times. Press and knead Guanyuan(RN4), Neiguan(PC6) and Zusanli(ST36) for 30 times respectively.

For patients with repeated hemoptysis, manual manipulation should be gentle and the time should be short. Massage is not advisable in the seizure of hemoptysis.

MEDICATED DIET

1. Soak *swallow's nest* 6 g and *white fungus* 9 g in clear water and wash them clean. Add *crystal sugar* 15 g in it and steam them over boiling water for oral administration. Take it twice to three times per week and 30 days consisted of one course.

2. Cut *radish* 500 g into pieces. Peel *apricot kernel* 15 g. Wash *pig's lung* 250 g clean and scald it in boiling water. Put three stuffs in an earthenware pot and simmer it till thoroughly done. Then season it with slat and eat the *pig's lung* and drink the soup.

3. Mix fresh *sheep's bile* 120 g and *honey* 250 g well. Steam it for two hours and reserve it in the bottle. Take 15 to 20 g each time in the morning and evening respectively.

QIGONG

Assume the stake – standing position. The whole body is relaxed. The two hands drop naturally to the lateral sides of the thighs. The tongue touches the upper palate. Baihui(DU20), Dantian and Huiyin(RN1) become a line. jTwo legs are slightly flexed. The feet separate the soulder's width and the foot tips are moved inwards.

With natural respiration, the mind should be concentrated on Yongquan(KI1) in the stake standing to let the point have the warm sensation (for about 3 minutes). In inhalation, the mind guides qi to rise from Yongquan(KI1) to Huiyin(RN1). Then guides qi along the Ren Channel to Dantian. In exhalation, the mind guides qi to go from Dantian along Huiyin(RN1) to Yongquan(KI1). Thus, with inhalation and exhalation, the circulation can be constantly repeated. It is advisable to practise it for 20 to 30 minutes each time.

PREVENTION

Keep regular life and change clothes according to the variation of weather so as to keep off exopathogens. Avoïd over intake of food greasy, sweet, pungent, sour salty, raw or cold so as to prevent the development of phlegm. Pain attention to physical training so as to build up health.

Chapter Eight
Asthma

Bronchial asthma is an allergic respiratory disease with recurrent attacks. Patients with asthma usually have a history of exudative conditions such as eczema, urticaria and angioneurotic edema. It is more commonly seen in children of four or five. Once they are exposed to allergens like bacterial or viral infection, flower powder, mites and dust, or after they take in fish, shrimps and protein, asthmatic attacks may occur. It may be often induced by sudden changes of the weather, overwork and mental irritation. Asthma is more common in spring and autumn, being prone to occur repeatedly. In infants and young children, it appears mostly like asthmatic bronchitis. With the growth of the children the frequency of attacks gradually reduces and the disease is even relieved. But when they grow older, the disease will reoccur. It is difficult to cure completely, usually becoming a life – long disorder.

ETIOLOGY AND PATHOGENESIS

Bronchial asthma results when exopathic factors act on the endopathic factors. The patient is generally weak in constitution and deficient in the functions of the lung, spleen and kidney. The deficiency of the lung may result in retention of water, the dysfunction of the spleen in water transportation, and deficiency of kidney in activating qi to promote diuresis. Retention and accumulation of water and dampness form turbid sputum, which stores in the interior. As a result, the sick child usually manifested by exudative conditions, showing pale complexion, fatness, recurrent eczema, loose muscle, and rumbling sound of the sputum in the throat, etc..

Because of the deficiency of lung – energy, the **yang** of the defensive function fails to strengthen the striae, which in turn makes one subject to attacks of exogenous pathogenic factors. In this case, if there are sudden changes of weather, the invasion of exopathogens into the body, the exposure to some substances, such as flower powder, mites, parasites and dust, irregular diet, over – eating of uncooked, cold, salty and acid food or taking in fish, shrimps and protein, the latent phlegm will be irritated, obstructing the air passage, making lung – qi unable to go up and down, therefore causing sudden attacks of asthma. Asthma that is due to retention of cold – type phlegm in the interior caused by the attack of wind – cold evil, internal injury by improper diet or deficiency of **yang** is known as cold – type asthma. Asthma that is due to deficiency of **yin** , accumulation of phlegm – heat in the lung or the transformation of cold – type phlegm into heat is known as heat – type asthma. If recurrent attacks of asthma further injure the vital essence of the lung, spleen and the kidney, the disease may present as deficient – type asthma with shortness of breath, bronchial wheezing when moving, and productive cough, which are commonly seen at the remission stage of the disease. Because the disease is caused by deficiency in origin and excess in superficiality, or a deficiency syndrome complicated with excess, it is difficult to be completely cured. When weather suddenly changes, diet is improper, and the mental irritated, the combination of exopathogens and endopathogens leads to recurrent attacks of asthma.

MAIN POINTS OF DIAGNOSIS

Bronchial asthma is divided into two different stages: attack and remission.

1. **Typical Attack:** It is marked by sudden onset or by the presymptoms of stuffy nose, sneezing, itching in the throat and oppressed feeling in the chest followed by asthma, shortness of breath, dyspnea, sound of sputum in thethroat, restlessness, failure of horizontal position, pale complexion, cyanosis of the lips and fingers, and cold sweat on the forehead. At beginning, there is dry cough, and later, the amount of sputum graduallyincreases. Once the sputum is removed, the attack will be relieved. The duration of the attack varies from a few minutes to several hours. A fewchildren are found in status asthmaticus.

2. **Signs:** Stethoscope examination finds obvious diminution of respiration in the two lungs, prolonged expiratory phase and wheezing all over the two lungs. In chronic patients, drumstick finger and barrel chest are commonly seen.

3. **X – ray Examination:** X – ray examination of the chest reveals changes ofemphysema. When secondary infection occurs, patchy shadows can be observed.

4. **Laboratory Test:** White cell count and neutrophilic granulocytesare generally normal; eosinophilic granulocytes increase by more than 5% ; whensecondary infection presents, white cell count and neutrophilic granulocytes mayincrease.

DIFFERENTIATION AND TREATMENT OF COMMONSYNDROMES

At the stage of an attack, it is dominated by excessivepathogenic factors. The suitable method is to relieve exterior syndrome, ventilatethe lung to resolve phlegm and relieve asthma. At the remission stage, it ischiefly characterized by deficiency of the lung, spleen and kidney. The method ofnourishing the lung, supporting the spleen and benefiting the kidney is applicableto strengthen the body resistance and or restore normal functioning of the body.

1. **Attack Stage**

1) **Asthma of Wind - cold Type.** Itcommonly occurs in cold seasons or when the patient is exposed to coldness.

Main Symptoms and Signs: Thetypical attack of asthma is manifested by cough with sputum whitish, clear, thin andfull of foam, no thirst, pale tongue with thin and whitish fur, and floating andtense pulse.

This syndrome is due to invasion of the lung by wind - cold. Theimpaired function of lung - qi in dispersing leads to coughing, nasal obstruction, sneezing and clear nasal discharge. The hidden phlegm and perverse qi combine tocause asthmatic breathing and gurgling with sputum. Thin and white sputum, awhite tongue coating, and a superficial and rolling pulse are all signs of cold andphlegm.

Therapeutic Principles: Ventilatingthe lung and dispelling cold, and alleviating asthma and cough.

Recipe: *Xiaoqinglong tang* (*Modified minor decoction of green dragon*)

Herba Ephedrae	4.5 g
Semen Armeniacae Amarum	6g
Rhizoma Pinelliae	6 g
Fructus Schisandrae	6 g
Flos Farfarae	6 g
Fructus Perillae	6 g
Semen Ginkgo	9 g
Cortex Mori Radicis	9 g
Lumbricus	9 g
Herba Houttuyniae	9 g
Radix Glycyrrhizae	3 g

Decoct the above ingredients in a right amount of water fororal administration.

Modification: If the heat pathogenaccumulates in the body, which is, at the same time, attacked by cold - pathogen, presenting as the syndrome of cold in superficies and heat in the interior, withfever, flushed face, red throat and thirst. *Radix Scutellariae* 9 g, *Radix Isalidis* 12 g and *Gypsum Fibrosum* 18 g should be added to clear away heat from the lung. If there is cough withproductive sputum, *Radix Peucedani* 9 g, *Bulbus Fritillariae Cirrhosae* 3 g and *RadixPlatycodi* 9 g should be added to relieve cough and resolvesputum. If asthma is severe, *Semen Raphani* 9 g, *Semen Sinapis Albae* 9 g and *FructusAurantii* 9 g should be added to alleviate asthma and cough.

2) **Asthma due to Phlegm – heat**

Main Symptoms and Signs: It ischaracterized by a typical attack with fullness sensation in the chest and heavybreath, thick and yellowish sputum, fever, flushed face, thirst with inclination todrink, yellow urine and dry stool, reddish tongue with yellowish fur, andsmooth and rapid pulse.

This syndrome is due to invasion of the lung by wind – heat or bycold which turns into heat. Heat condenses body fluid into phlegm, which blocksair passage and impairs the lung's function in dispersing with the ensuingsymptoms of coughing, with thick and yellow sputum, and asthmatic breathing. Thirst, inflamed throat, a red tongue tip with yellow and sticky coating, and a rollingand rapid pulse are all signs of retention of phlegm heat in the interior.

Therapeutic Principles: Clearingaway heat pathogen and eliminating sputum.

Recipe: *Jiajian dingchuan tang* (*Modified decoction for relieving asthma*)

Herba Ephedrae	6 g
Semen Ameniacae Amarum	3 g
Gypsum Fibrosum	15 g
Radix Scutellariae	9 g
Fructus Aurantii	9 g
Cortex Mori Radicis	12 g
Semen Lepidii seuDescurainiae	6 g
Fructus PerillaePraeparata	9 g
Rhizoma Pinelliae	9 g

Decoct the above ingredients in a right amount of water fororal administration.

Modification: If there is highfever, *Flos Lonicerae* 12 g and *Radix Bupleuri* 12 g should be addedto clear away the heat pathogen; if associated with yellowish thick sputum, *Fructus Trichosanthis* 9 g, *SemenRaphani* 9 g and *Radix Trichosanthis*9 g should be added to clear away heat and resolve sputum.

3) **Type of Excess in the Upper and Deficiency in the Lower**

Main Symptoms and Signs: Frequentrelapse of asthma which is even protracted, rale like snore in the throat, profuse sputum, fullness in the chest, weakness in coughing, pale or even livid complexion, sweating, cold limbs, purplishdark tongue with whitish greasy coating, and deep thready pulse.

Therapeutic Principles: Checkingupward adverse flow of qi to relieve asthma, warming the kidney to improveinspiration.

Recipe: *Suzi jiangqi tang*(*Decoction of Perilla seed for descending qi*)

Fructus Perillae	9 g
Cortex Magnoliae Officinalis	9 g
Radix Peucedani	9 g
Rhizoma Pinelliae	9 g
Radix Angelicae Sinensis	9 g
Pericarpium Citri Reticulatae	9 g
Cortex Cinnamomi	4.5 g
Radix Glycyrrhizae	4.5 g
Rhizoma Zingiberis Recens	3 pieces

Decoct the above ingredients in a right amount of water fororal administration.

Modification: In case of asthmawhich is severe in the posture of lying down, and edema of the face and limbs, thedrugs added are *Semen Lepidii seu Descurainiae* 15g, *Cortex Mori* 12 g, *Semen Plantaginis* 15 g.

In case of deficiency of qi, the drugs added are*Radix Codonopsis* 15 g and *Fructus Schisandrae*6 g.

In case of deficiency of yang, the drugsadded are Radix Aconiti Lateralis Praeparata 9 g and*Semen Juglandis* 15 g.

2. **Remission Stage**

1) **Deficiency ofQi in Lung and Spleen**

Main Symptoms and Signs: Itis characterized by emaciation, pale complexion, weak breath, poor appetite, listlessness, asthenia, cough with abundant clear, thin and whitish expectoration, rumbling sound of the sputum in the throat or occasional mild asthma, pale tonguewith whitish fur, fine and slow pulse.

TherapeuticPrinciples: Invigorating the spleen and benefiting qi, and resolving phlegm andrelieving cough.

Recipe: *Renshenwuweizi tang*(*Decoction of Codonopsis Pilosula and Schisandra*)

Radix CodonopsisPilosulae	9 g
Radix Astragali seuHedysari	9 g
Rhizoma AtractylodisMacrocephalae	9 g
Poria	9 g
Fructus Schisandrae	6 g
Cortex Mori Radicis	9 g
Bulbus FritillariaeCirrhosae	3 g
Pericarpium CitriReticulatae	6 g

Rhizoma Pinellae 6 g
Radix Ophiopogonis 9 g
Radix Glycyrrhizae 3 g

Decoct the above ingredients in a right amount of water fororal administration.

Modification: If the patient haspoor appetite and feels abdominal distention, *Massa FermentataMedicinalis* 9 g, *Fructus Hordei Germinatus*9 g, *Fructus Amomi* 3 g and *Rhizoma Dioscoreae* 6 g should beadded to invigorate the spleen and improve appetite; if there are abundant thinexpectoration, whitish and greasy or whitish and smooth fur on the tongue, modified *Erchen tang* should be used toresolve sputum and relieve cough, which is composed of *PericarpiumCitri Reticulatae* 6 g, *Poria* 9 g, *Rhizoma Pinelliae* 9 g, *Bulbus Fritillariae Cirrhosae* 3 g, *Cortex Mori Radicis* 12 g and *Radix Glycyrrhizae* 3 g.

Deficiency of both the Lung and Kidney

Main Symptoms and Signs: It ismanifested by pale complexion, cold extremities, aversion to cold, spontaneoussweating, cough with abundant sputum or asthma of insufficiency type, anorexia, shortness of breath, pale tongue with whitish fur, and fine and faint pulse.

Therapeutic Principles: Improvinginspiration by warming the kidney and invigorating the lung to relieve asthma.

Recipe: *Jiajian jingui shenqiwan (Modified golden bolus for promoting kidney – qi)*

Radix Aconiti 6 g
Rhizoma RehmanniaePraeparata 9 g
Fructus Corni 6 g
Rhizoma Dioscoreae 6 g
Fructus Schisandrae 6 g
Poria 9 g
Cortex Moutan Radicis 9 g
Juglandis Regiae 9 g
Radix CondonopsisPilosulae 9 g
Radix Glycyrrhizae 3 g

Decoct the above ingredients in a right amount of water fororal administration.

OTHER THERAPIES

1. Simple Recipe and Proved Prescription

1) Lumbricus, which is made into fine powder afterbeing baked dry for oral dose, three times a day, 1 – 3 g a time, taken before meal. This recipe has an effect of clearing away heat and resolving phlegm, andtranquilizing the mind. It is suitable for the attack stage of asthma.

2) The powder of placenta, orally, 3 – 5 g a time, 3 times daily. It is effective in increasing resistance against diseases and preventingrecurrence. It is applicable to remission stage of asthma.

3) *Juglandis Regiae* 9 g, *Cordyceps* 9 g and *Gecko* 9 g, which are usedseparately or in combination. They have an effect of tonifying the kidney to astringe thelung and is suitable for the remission stage of asthma.

2. Acupuncture and Moxibustion

1) Body Acupuncture: When asthma attacks, insert needles into theacupoints of Dingchuan(EX – B1), Tiantu(RN22) and Danshu(BL19) with rapid turning movementsor keep the needles in for 15 minutes once daily.

3. Application Method

1) *Semen Sinapis Albae* 15 g, *Herba Asari* 2 g, *Rhizoma Corydalis* 9 g and *Radix Euphorbiae Kansui* 9 g are allmade into powder, mixed together with some *Succus Zingiberis* and then shaped into six drug cakes with a small amount of *Moschus* or *Flos Syzygii powder* put inside each of them. They are applied on acupoints ofBaliao(BL31 – 34), Feishu(BL13) andGaohuang(BL43).

Direction: During the midsummer theapplication is carried out once every 10 days, three times a course, each timelasting two hours. This therapy is carried on for 3 years. It is suitable for theremission stage of asthma and effective to reduce and relieve the attack ofasthma.

2) **External Application of Herbal Preparations**

This method is recommended in the treatment ofasthma at the remission stage. 30 g of *Semen Sinapis Albae*, 30 g of *Rhizoma Corydalis*, 15 g of *Herba Asari* and 15 g of *Radix Euphorbiae Kansui* are groundinto powder, which is made into 6 medicinal cakes with a proper amount of freshginger juice. 3 g of *Powder of Moschus* or *Powder of Flos Caryophylli* areplaced into the centre of these cakes. They are then applied onto Bailao (EX), which is one *cun* lateral and 2 *cun* aboveDazhui (DU14), Feishu (BL13) andGaohuangshu(BL43) on both sides. This treatmentis given once every five days in winter and spring, and once every ten days insummer, three times successively. The cakes are retained on these points for twohours each time, or for only 20 minutes, if ionization is introduced. Generally, the local area will become congested or flushed after the removal of the cakes. Blisters may occur in a few patients. *Gentian violet* is smeared if theblisters are broken.

3) There is another method of external application: 3 g of *Semen Sinapis Albae*, 0.6 g of *Herba Asari*, 1 g of *pepper* and 1 g of *Rhizoma Typhonii* are all groundinto powder, which is applied to Feishu(**BL**13) after being mixed with *ginger juice*. The preparation isapplied before bed time and removed the next morning. If there is strong reactionin the local area, the preparation can be retained on the point for one to twohours. The treatment is given every day or every two day, seven sessionsconsisted of one course.

Massage Therapy

1) **First, pushing manipulation is preferable, pushing transversely the chest and abdominal regions mainly on the acupoints ofHuagai**(**RN**20) and Danzhong(**RN**17) in turn, the lumbodorsalregions (from the above downward, mainly Feishu(**BL**13), Geshu(**BL**17) and Mingmen(**DU**4) and spinal column and itsbilateral sides, and then press Feishu(**BL**13) and Geshu(**BL**17) once every one to two days, 10 times a course, which is suitable for remission stage.

2) Slowly push withone finger from Taintu(**RN**22) to Danzhong(**RN**17) to and fro repeatedly for 2to 3 minutes. Then push with two fingers from Danzhong(**RN**17)to the bilateral sides for 200 to 300 times; lift and grasp the neckfor one to two minutes. Then flatly push the chest and back; obliquely push thetwo costal regions till the heat penetrates; press and push Feishu(**BL**13) and Geshu(**BL**13) till there are soreness and distension; lift andgrasp Jianjing(**GB**21) for 3 to 5 times; flatly pushthe upper arm and forearm and then lift and grasp them andHegu(**LI**4); pull the fingers; rub and shake the upperlimbs; rotate the shoulders forwards and backwards for 3 circles respectively.

MEDICATED DIET

1. Decoct 6 g of *ephedra*, 6 g of *dried ginger* and 3 g of *licorice root* first and strain thedregs out of the decoction. Then add 100 g of *polishedround - grained rice* and proper amount of water to make gruel; finallyscatter the *sliced Chinese green onion* intogruel when it is done. Take it twice a day. It can be used as an auxillarytreatment for asthma of cold type.

1. Decoct 30 g of *gypsum*, 21 g of *bitter apricot kernel*, 15 g of *peucedanum root* and 9 g of *licorice root* together in waterfirst and sift out 500 ml of the decoction; then

add 100 g of *waxgourd slice*, 150 g of *crystalsugar*, 100 g of *smashed Sichuan fritillary bulb*, 30g of powder of *red tangerine peel*, 6 pieces of *peeled and pounded pears* andproportional amount of alum solution. Mix them well and steam the mixture in the bowlover the boiling water for about 50 minutes until it becomes sticky and thickextract. Take the extract in several days. It is suitable to asthma of heat type.

QIGONG

Assume the sitting or standing posture. Breatheevenly and relax the whole body. First push with the palmar sides of the index, ring and little fingers from the sternal notch down to the xiphoid process for 36times; then knead Danzhong(**RN**17) between the two breasts withthe palmar sides of the four fingers for 36 times. Breathe naturally and focusthe mind beneath the hands. When exhaling, push with the right palm from themedian line of the chest to the left side for 5 to 10 times; pause when inhaling. Dofor 10 breaths altogether. Then push with the left palm from the median line ofthe chest to the right side for 10 breaths. The mind follows the hand. Whenexhaling, rub and knead with the flat palms from the armpits to the bilateral sidesof the abdomen respectively for 5 to 10 times.

PREVENTION AND NURSING

1. The patient should do physical exercise andbuild up health so as to reduce the attack of the disease.

2. Active preventive measures should be taken against thediseases related with asthma, such as tonsillitis, decayed teeth, nasosinusitis andpneumonia, and proper treatment must be given when any of them occurs.

3. The sick child should keep a regular diet and a regular dailylife, refraining from sour, salty, cold and uncooked food. He must avoid suddenchanges of the temperature and the weather, keeping away from the sensitinogenthat will induce asthma.

4. When asthma attacks, the sick child should be kept quiet toavoid psychological tense. When necessary, oxygen should be given, and a quietroom with fresh air is also helpful.

5. At the remission stage, medicinal herbs with the function ofstrengthening the body resistance should be used to reduce the recurrence orrelieve the symptoms of the disease.

6. Find out the anaphylactogen and do the best to avoid inhaling, touching or taking it again. Conditions permitting, desensitization treatmentmay be performed with the ex-

tract of anaphylactogen.

7. In daily life, strike a proper balance between work and rest, prevent the infection of the upper respiratory tract, give up smoking and limitalcohol drinking, and keep off emotional stimulation.

DISCUSSION

Asthma at the acute stage is usually of theexcess type. Cold and heat must be differentiated. Asthma due to cold ischaracterized by clear nasal discharge, thin, white and frothy sputum, and a white tonguecoating, while asthma due to heat is marked by dryness of the nose with turbid andyellow discharge, thick and yellowish - white sputum, inflamed throat, a redremission stage is often of the deficiency type. It is necessary to make clear whichof the three organs is deficient, the lung, spleen or kidney. Of the three, deficiency of the lung qi is the most common, and then the deficiency of spleen qiand deficiency of kidney qi.

During the acute stage, the patient should be kept quiet andcalm. The air in the room must be fresh, and simple and less salty food isrecommended. During the remission stage, the patient should eat better food, be exposedto more sunshine, and do proper exercises to build up health. Care should betaken not to catch cold when weather changes. Such areas as Tiantu(**RN**22), Bailao(**EX - HN**)and Feishu(**BL**13) should be kept warm all thetime.

Chapter Nine
Chronic Rhinitis

Chronic rhinitis is a chronic inflammatory change of the nasal mucosa, mainly due to the protraction of acute rhinitis. Its main symptom is nasal obstruction. This disease is called *bi zhi* (nasal obstruction) in traditional Chinese medicine.

MAIN POINTS OF DIAGNOSIS

1. The nasal obstruction is either alternate, intermittent or continuous.

2. The nasal mucosa swells or becomes thick, especially that of the inferior nasal concha.

3. Hyposmia is fluctuating.

4. There is pain and itching in the throat and tinnitus or hypoacusis may occur.

DIFFERENTIATION AND TREATMENT OF COMMON SYNDROMES

1. Internal Treatment

1) Qi-deficiency of both the Lung and Spleen

Main Symptoms and Signs: The nasal obstruction is relieved in the morning and aggravated at night and becomes severe if exposed to cold. When the patient lies in lateral recumbent position, it is less severe in the upper part than in the lower one, or becomes alternate. The inferior nasal concha swells and has slight congestion. The conchae may contract if vasoconstrictor is used. There may be accompanying cough with thin sputum, short breath and asthenia. The tongue is light red, its fur white and the pulse moderate.

Therapeutic Principles: Strengthening the spleen, warming the lung, removing cold and clearing away the obstruction from the upper orifices.

Recipe: *Pill for warming the lung to stop running nose with additional ingredients*

Radix Ginseng	6-9 g
Herba Schizonepetae	9 g
Fructus Chebulae	9 g
Radix Platycodi	9 g
Otolith Pseudosciaenae	15 g
Radix Angelicae Dahuricae	15 g

Herba Asari (decocted later) 3 g
Radix Glycyrrhizae 6 g
Radix Astragali seu Hedysari 24 g

Decoct the above ingredients in a right amount of water for oral administration.

Stagnation of Qi and Blood Stasis

Main Symptoms and Signs: The patient has continuous nasal obstruction and hyposmia. The inferior nasal concha is hypertrophic and dark red or like moruloid and insensitive to vasoconstrictor. There are accompanying symptoms such as dizziness, a feeling of fullness in the ear and hypoacusis. The tongue is red or has petechiae on it. The pulse is taut and uneven.

Therapeutic Principles: Promoting blood circulation to remove blood stasis and resolving masses to clear away obstruction from the upper orifices.

Recipe: *Peach kernel and Safflower decoction of four ingredients, compounded with Xanthium Powder*

Semen Persicae 9 g
Flos Carthami 9 g
Radix Rehmanniae 9 g
Fructus Xanthii 9 g
Herba Menthae 9 g
Flos Magnoliae 9 g
Radix Angelicae Sinensis 15 g
Radix Paeoniae Rubra 15 g
Rhizoma Ligustici Chuanxiong 12 g
Radix Angelicae Dahuricae 18 g

Decoct the above ingredients in a right amount of water for oral administration.

For those with severe nasal obstruction, add 9 grams of *Spina Gleditsiae* and 9 grams of *Squama Manitis*. For those with headache, add 9 grams of *Rhizoma et Radix Ligustici* and 9 grams of *Fructus Viticis*. For those who have severe blood stasis, add 9 grams of *Rhizoma Sparganii* and 9 grams of *Rhizoma Zedoariae*. For those who have short breath and asthenia, add 15 grams of *Radix Codonopsis Pilosulae*, 9 grams of *Rhizoma Atractylodis Macrocephalae* and 9 grams of *Fructus Amomi*.

3) **Yin Deficiency of the Lung and Kidney**

Main Symptoms and Signs: Dryness and a sensation of obstruction in the nose, hyposmia, blood threads in the nasal discharge, fetor narium, dry throat, dry cough with little sputum, feverish sensation in the palms and soles. Red tongue with little coating, thready and rapid pulse.

Chronic Rhinitis

Therapeutic Principles: Nourish the lung and replenish the kidney.

Recipe:

Dried rehmannia root	15 g
Lily bulb	15 g
Scrophularia root	12 g
Ophiopogon root	12 g
Fritillary bulb	9 g
Platycodon root	9 g
Moutan bark	9 g
Peppermint	6 g
Licorice root	6 g

4) **Acumulated Heat in the Lung Meridian**

Main Symptoms and Signs: Profuse yellow turbid nasal discharge, long duration of nasal obstruction, hyposmia, dizziness, distension in the head, hypomnesia. Red tongue with yellow coating, wiry and thready pulse.

Therapeutic Principles: Clear away heat, promote the dispersing function of the lung and open the orifice.

Recipe:

Xanthium	9 g
Magnolia flower	9 g
Anemarrhena rhizome	9 g
Cimicifuga rhizome	9 g
Peppermint	6 g
Capejasmine fruit	12 g
Lily bulb	15 g
Loquat leaf	12 g
Gypsum	30 g
Dahurian angelica root	15 g

2. **External Treatment**

1) Use *Effectual Nose Drops* for nasal drip. It should be done three times a day.

2) Blow *Powder of Eardust of Yellow Croaker* into the nasal cavity. Its ingredients are:

Otolith Pseudosciaenae	9 g
Borneolum Syntheticum	0.9 g
Flos Magnoliae	6 g
Herba Asari	3 g

All the above drugs are to be pounded into powder and blown into the nose three times a day.

3) **Massage the nasal part**

Knead with two thumbs to and fro along the back of the nose until a sensation of enough heat is produced. Do this twice a day.

4) **Simple and Convenient Recipe**

Add a little borneol into some sesame oil and use the mixture for nasal drip three times daily. It is suitable for the patients with yin deficiency of both lung and kidney.

ACUPUNCTURE AND MOXIBUSTION

1. Body Acupuncture

Main Points: Yingxiang(LI20), Yintang(EX-HN3), Lieque(LU7), Hegu(LI4), Fengmen(BL12), and Dazhui(DU14).

Complementary Points: Add Taiyang(EX-HN5) for headache.

Method: Use the filiform needles to puncture the points with even movement. Retain the needles for 30 minutes.

2. Auricular Acupuncture

Prescribed Points: Neibi(TG_4) internal nose, E(AT_1) forehead, and Fei(CO_{14}) lung.

Method: Puncture the points with filiform needles and retain them for 20 minutes. The seed-embedding method or subcutaneous needle is also applicable.

MASSAGE

Press and knead Baihui(DU20), Shangxing(DU23), Yintang(EX-HN3) and Yingxiang (LI20) for 30 times respectively. Chafe along the sides of the nose for 30 times. Rub the hands and wash the face for 50 times. Grasp and knead Hegu(LI4) of both sides for 30 times respectively and pinch Shaoshang(LU11) for 20 times.

MEDICATED DIET

1. Have one duck rid of its feathers and internal organs. Put the duck, with 15 g of *Chinese caterpillar fungus* in its belly, in a plate with just the right amount of water. Steam it over the boiling water until the duck is done. Take the duck and soup.

2. Cook gruel with 60 g of *polished round-grained rice*, 20 g of *mung bean* and

15 g of *lily bulb*. Add some crystal sugar just as the gruel is half done. Take one dose a day for 10 days totally.

QIGONG

1. Wash the face

Two hands are rubbed hot, then the middle fingers rub the lateral sides of the nose upwards with other fingers; while reaching the forehead, the hands separate and rub two cheeks downwards. It can be repeated for 9 times. This section can promote the smooth flow of qi and blood on the face and prevent common cold. **2. Rub the nose**

The index fingers are piled up on the middle fingers. The middle fingers are pressed on the lateral sides of the nose to rub the nose upwards and downwards. Then the thumb knuckles are placed on Yingxiang(LI20) bilateral to the nose to knead them for 20 times. The section can prevent common cold and unobstruct the nasal cavity.

Chapter Ten
Allergic Rhinitis

Allergic rhinitis is an alleric disease caused by the sensitinogen acting on the mucous membranes of the nasal cavity, also called perennial allergic rhinitis. Clinically it has the following features: itching in the nose, sneeze, watery nasal discharge, nasal obsruction coming and going suddenly. It is called *bi qiu* in traditional Chinese medicine, a reference to allergic rhinits.

MAIN POINTS OF DIAGNOSIS

1. Itching in the nasal cavity occurs suddenly, accompanied with itching in the eyes and pharynx.

2. The patient has one sneeze after another, sometimes dozens of them in succession.

3. There is watery nasal discharge with foams. In the period of acute reaction, plenty of nasal discharge comes out continuously.

4. At the beginning the nasal obstruction is transient. Then it becomes continuous, or accompanied with hyposmia.

5. The mucous membrane in the nasal cavity (chiefly in the middle and inferior conchae) shows swelling, pale or greyish blue in color, and moist and pliable. During the course, moruloid change in the inferior concha or a polypoid change in the middle concha will occur, with a lot of watery secretion in the nasal meatus.

DIFFERENTIATION AND TREATMENT OF COMMON SYNDROMES

1. Internal Treatment

1) **Deficiency of Spleen Qi**

Main Symptoms and Signs: The patient has paroxysmal itching, sore and swelling in the nose, sneezes with much watery nasal dicharge, intermittent nasal obstruction and pale nasal mucosa with local swelling, accompanied with tiredness or asthenia, deficiency in breath and no desire for talking, poor appetite, loose stool, aversion to cold and cool limbs, sore in the loins and frequent urination at night. The tongue is light red, with thin and white fur and the pulse is thready.

Therapeutic Principles: Strengthening the spleen, replenishing qi and dispersing pathogenic cold to remove ovstruction from the upper orifices.

Recipe: *Decoction for reinforcing middle – jiao and replenishing qi compounded with Xanthium Powder*

Radix Angelicae Sinensis	9 g
Radix Ginseng	9 g
Radix Astragali seu Hedysari	18 g
Fructus Xanthii	9 g
Flos Magnoliae	9 g
Herba Menthae	9 g
Rhizoma Cimicifugae	9 g
Pericarpium Citri Reticulatae	9 g
Rhizoma Atractylodis Macrocephalae	9 g
Radix Glycyrrhizae Praeparata	9 g
Radix Bupleuri	9 g
Radix Angelicae Dahuricae	15 g

Decoct the above ingredients in a right amount of water for oral administration.

For those with apparent manifestations of deficiency of the lung – qi, increase the dsage of *Radix Astragali seu Hedysari* to 30 grams and add 9 grams of *radix Ledebouriellae* to the recipe. For those with accompanying abdominal distension and loose stool, add 15 grams of *Semen Dolichoris Album* and 18 grams of *Semen Coicis*. For those with soreness in the loins and frequent urination at night, add 6 grams of *Rhizoma Curculiginis*, 9 grams of *Radix Aconiti Praeparata* or use *Golden Chamber bolus for Tonifying Kidney – qi* (recorded by the book entitled ***Synopsis of Prescription of Golden Chamber***). For those who have hypertrophic inferior nasal concha, add 15 grams of *Radix Paeoniae Rubra*, 9 grams of *Rhizoma Ligustici Chuanxiong* and 9 grams of *Fructus Liquidambaris*. For those who have plenty of watery nasal discharge, add 9 grams of *Fructus Schisandrae*, 9 grams of *Fructus Mume* and 3 grams of *Herba Asari*.

2) **Attack by Pathogenic Wind**

Main Symptoms and Signs: Paroxysmal itching, sore and distending sensation in the nose, sneezes with much watery nasal discharge, accompanied by cough, a little sputum, sore throat and headache. Red tongue with thin and white coating, floating pulse.

Therapeutic Principles: Expel wind and open the upper orifice.

Recipe:

Mulberry leaf	9 g
Bitter apricot kernel	9 g

Platycodon root 6 g
Xanthium 9 g
Magnolia flower 9 g
Dahurian angelica root 15 g
Ledebouriella root 9 g
Licorice root 3 g

3) **Deficiency of Lung Qi**

Main Symptoms and Signs: Intermittent nasal obstruction, pale nasal mucosa with local swelling, accompanied by shortness of breath, no desire for talking, poor appetite, tiredness, aversion to cold and cold limbs. Pale tongue with thin and white coating, thready pulse.

Therapeutic Principles: Strengthen the lung and replenish qi and open the upper orifice.

Recipe:

Astragalus root 30 g
Dried rehmannia root 12 g
Ophiopogon root 15 g
Fritillary bulb 9 g
Dendrobium 15 g
Adenophora root 15 g
Peppermint 6 g
Cimicifua rhizome 9 g
Prepared licorice 6 g

External Treatment

1) Blow *Biyun powder* into the nose. Its ingredients are:

Herba Centipedae 30 g
Rhizoma Ligustici Chuanxiong 30 g
Flos Magnoliae 6 g
Herba Asari 6 g
Indigo Naturalis 3 g

Grind the above drugs together into fine powder and blow it into the nose three times a day.

2) Insert into the nose *Ointment Tablet of Eardust of Yellow Croaker*. The ingredients are as follows:

Otolith Pseudosciaenae 9 g
borneolum Syntheticum 0.9 g

Flos Magnoliae	6 g
Herba Asari	3 g

Grind the above drugs together into fine powder and add quantum sufficit of vaseline to make *ointment tablets* from it. Insert one *ointment tablet* in the nose each day.

ACUPUNCTURE AND MOXIBUSTION

1. Body Acupuncture

Main Points: Lieque(**LU**7), Hegu(**LI**4), Yingxiang(**LI**20), and Yintang(**EX-HN**3).

Complementary Points: Add Taiyang(**EX-HN**5) for headache.

Method: Apply the filiform needles with sedation and retain the needles for 15 minutes, and manipulate them once or twice in interval.

2. Auricular Acupuncture

Prescribed Points: Neibi(TG_4) internal nose, E(AT_1) forehead, Fei(CO_{14}) lung, Shenshangxian(TG_{2p}) adrenal gland.

Method: 2 - 3 points are selected each time. The filiform needles are applied with strong stimulation and retained for 30 minutes. The seed-embedding method or subcutaneous needle is also applicable.

MASSAGE

Press and knead Fengchi(**GB**20), Fengmen(**BL**12), Taiyang(**EX-HN**5) and Yintang (**EX-HN**1) for 30 times respectively. Push the forehead divergently for 30 times. Rub the hands to wash the face 30 times. Knead Danzhong(**RN**17) 30 times. Scrub Dazhui(**DU**14) for 30 times and press and knead Hegu(**LI**4) for 30 times.

MEDICATED DIET

Wash 50 g of *polished round-grained rice* and put it in a cooking pot. Add right amount of water and heat it over a strong fire until it boils. Then boil it over a gentle fire for 40 minutes. Put in 50 g of *lily bulbs* and go on cooking until it is done. Add crystal sugar before eating. Take the gruel once in the morning and in the evening respectively.

QIGONG

Assume the sitting or standing posture. Get rid of nasal discharge. Relax and tranquilize the body naturally and breathe evenly. Rub the dorsa of both thumbs against each other until they are warm. Then slightly rub the two sides of the nose. Rub 5 times in inhalation and 5 times in exhalation. Do 6 breaths altogether.

Press the tip of the middle finger of the right hand on the apex of the nose. Move leftward in circular motion for 5 times in inhalation and rightward for 5 times in exhalation. Do 6 times altogether.

Chapter Eleven
Infantile Pneumonia

Pneumonia is a very common disease, especially in infants. It is usually defined as acute inflammation of the lung caused by bacteria, viruses, *Mycoplasma pneumoniae*, etc. clinically it can be classified as pneumococcal pneumonia, staphylococcal pneumonia, adenoviral pneumonia and so on, and pathogenically, as lobar pneumonia, lobular pneumonia, interstitial pneumonia and bronchopneumonia. This disease belongs to the categories of *mapi feng*(acute infantile pneumonia), *bao chuan* (sudden attack of asthma) in traditional Chinese medicine.

ETIOLOGY AND PATHOGENESIS

Children are weak in constitution and qi, delicate in **Zang** and **Fu**, so that the superficial qi fails to protect the body against disease. If the wind – pathogen invades the lung through the mouth and nose, causing obstruction of the lung – qi and dysfunction of water fluid transportation, blocking of the air passage by the accumulated sputum, there will be followed by cough, shortness of breath, rale in the throat, etc.. If the warm – pathogens invades the lung, burns the fluids and makes them into sputum, and in turn, the sputum – heat obstructs the air passage, high fever will occur with excessive thirst, and productive cough, etc.. The disease may continues to involve other viscera. The obstruction of the lung – qi may affect the circulation of the heart – blood. If there exist the stasis of blood flow, malnutrition of the heart and stagnation of liver – qi, the disease may present as deteriorated case with cyanosis of mouth and nails, dark – purplish tongue and enlargement of the liver. Failure of vital energy against pathogenic factor, stagnation of heart – blood and insufficiency of the heart – yang result in sudden prostration syndrome, manifested as pale complexion, dyspnea, restlessness, cold limbs, excessive perspiration, etc.. If the stagnation of the lung – qi is severe, it will affect the function of the spleen and stomach, marked by poor appetite, abdominal distention and constipation. Because the lung is responsible for inspiration and the kidney governs the reception of air, the lung acts as the master of air, and the kidney, the root of it. Stagnation of the lung – qi for long will certainly affect the kidney which refuses to recept the air, resulting in hypopnea, cacorhythm or respiration like sighing or weeping. This is the dangerious sign of respiratory failure. If the pathogenic heat is too high which invades the interior of Jueyin, there appear high fever, coma, convulsion, etc..

In the later stages of pneumonia in children, it is chiefly manifested by consumption of qi and yin, with the lingering of pathogenic factor due to weakened body resistance, deficiency of the lung and spleen, and the lung – heat caused by yin deficiency.

MAIN POINTS OF DIAGNOSIS

1. Upper respiratory tract infection, characterized by fever, cough and nasal discharge, is followed by symptoms and signs of pneumonia, such as tachypnea, dyspnea, cyanosis, pallor, nares flaring, 3 concave signs and restlessness, which may be accompanied with vomiting, abdominal distention, tachycardia and hepatomegaly.

2. Physical examinations may reveal dullness in the affected area through percussion, and diminished breathing sound, fine cracking rales or crepitus and moist rales on the affected side through auscultation.

3. Laboratory examinations may show elevated leukocyte count in the cases with bacterial pneumonia. Bacteriological evidence may be found by cultures and isolation of bacteria from the sputum, tracheal aspirates, and pleural fluid obtained through thoracentesis.

4. Pneumonographic changes in early pneumonia include consolidation, pleural reaction with the presence of fluid, roughened lung – marking and sporadic mottlings on the lower field of the lung. It is very important that roentgenographic demonstration of complete resolution should be obtained 3 – 4 weeks after disappearance of symptoms.

DIFFERENTIATION AND TREATMENT OF COMMON SYNDROMES

1. Wind – cold Pathogen Tightening the Lung

Main Symptoms and Signs: Aversion to cold, fever, anhidrosis, absence of thirst, cough with unclear throat, white and thin sputum, normal tongue proper with thin and white or white and greasy fur, floating, tight and rapid pulse, and blue red superficial venule of the index finger existing more often on the wind pass.

Invasion of the lung by wind – cold via the skin and hair leads to blockage of air passage and upward disturbance of lung – qi. This explains coughing, shortness of breath and thin and white sputum. Invasion of the body surface by wind – cold inhibits defensive yang, in which condition, yang – qi is not able to be distributed throughout the body, and the symptoms or aversion to cold, fever and absence of sweating will lollow. A thin and white or white and sticky tongue coating, and a superficial, tense and rapid pulse are all the signs of invasion of the lung by wind – cold.

Therapeutic Principles: Relieving exterior syndrome with drugs pungent in flavor and warm in property, ventilating the lung and climinating sputum.

Recipe: *Modified huagai powder*

Herba Ephedrae	6 g
Semen Armeniacae Amarum	6 g
Fructus Perillae	6 g
Pericarpium Citri Reticulatae	6 g
Rhizoma Pinelliae	6 g
Radix Asteris	9 g
Flos Farfarae	9 g
Rhizoma Zingiberis Recens	1 slice
Fructus Ziziphi Jujubae	5 pieces

Decoct the above ingredients in a right amount of water for oral administration.

Besides, in case of abundant expectoration, 6 grams of *Semen Raphani* and 6 grams of *Semen Sinapis Albae* should be included. For those with cold – syndrome in both exterior and interior, 1.5 grams of *Herba Asari* should be added.

2. **Wind – heat Pathogen Tightening the Lung**

Main Symptoms and Signs: Fever with sweat, thirst, cough with thick sputum, rapid breath with nares flaring, red face and lips, reddish throat, yellow urine, constipation or mucous stool, red tongue with yellowish fur, floating and rapid or smooth and rapid pulse, and blue purple superficial venule of the index finger existing more often on the qi pass.

This syndrome results from invasion of the lung by wind – cold which turns into heat, or from direct invasion by heat. Thus the function of the lung in descending is impaired, and symptoms of fever and thirst will ensue. Heat condenses body fluid into phlegm, which explains sticky and yellow sputum. Since the throat is the gateway of the lung and stomach, invasion of the lung by wind – heat will give rise to inflamed and sore throat. The combination of phlegm and heat is the cause of coughing and ala nasi trembling. A red tongue with thin and yellow coating, and a superficial, rolling and rapid pulse are both signs of wind – heat.

Therapeutic Principles: Relieving exterior syndrome with drugs pungent in flavor and cool in property, ventilating the lung and eliminating sputum.

Recipe: *Decoction of Ephedra, Apricot kernel, Gypsum and Licorice with additional ingredients*

Semen Armeniacae Amarum	6 g
Gypsum Fibrosum	18 g
Radix Glycyrrhizae	3 g

Flos Lonicerae 12 g
Radix Scutellariae 9 g
Herba Houttuyniae 9 g
Radix Isatidis 9 g
Radix Platycodi 9 g

Decoct the above ingredients in a right amount of water for oral administration.

Besides, in case of severe cough, add 12 grams of *Cortex Mori Radicis* and 9 grams of *Flos Lonicerae*. For those with high fever and constipation, add 15 grams of *Rhizoma Phragmitis* and 20 ml of *Succus Bambusae* which is to be mixed up with the finished decoction.

3. Stagnation of Phlegm – heat in the Lung

Main Symptoms and Signs: High fever, vexation, accumulation of phlegm in throat, polypnea, dyspnea, nares flaring even flaring of the hypochondria, abnormal protrusion of the chest and elevation of the shoulders, shaking of the body and plucking of the abdomen in severe cases, constipation, oliguria with yellow urine, red tongue with yellow and dry fur, full, slippery and rapid pulse, and blue purple superficial venule of the index finger existing more often on the qi pass.

This syndrome is due to blockage of the collateral of the lung with phlegm – heat. Upward movement of phlegm along with perverse qi is the cause of high fever, coughing, asthmatic breathing and gurgling with sputum. The blockage of air passage by phlegm – heat gives rise to shortness of breath and ala nasi trembling, or even cyanosis of lips. Constipation, a red tongue with yellow coating, and a rolling and rapid pulse are all signs of phlegm – heat.

Therapeutic Principles: Clearing away pathogenic heat, ventilating the lung and eliminating phlegm to relieve asthma.

Recipe: *Modified prescriptin of five – tiger decoction and decoction of Lepidium seed and Chinese – date for removing phlegm from the lung*

Herba Ephedrae 6 g
Semen Armeniacae Amarum 9 g
Gypsum Fibrosum (To be decocted first) 30 g
Herba Asari 6 g
Radix Glycyrrhizae 3 g
Semen Lepidii seu Descurainiae 9 g
Fructus Ziziphi Jujubae 5 pieces
Concretio Silicea Bambusae 9 g
Radix Scutellariae 9 g

Arisaema cum Bile 9 g
Herba Houttuyniae 12 g
Succus bambosae 20 ml

Bamboo juice is taken after being infused in the finished decoction.

Decoct the above ingredients in a right amount of water for oral administration.

Besides, 3 grams of *Radix et Rhizoma Rhei* which is to be decocted later should be added in case of constipation and abdominal distention. For those with severe cyanosis, remove *Apricot kernel*, add 12 grams of *Radix Salviae Miltiorrhizae*, 9 grams of *Radix Paeoniae Rubra*, 6 grams of *Flos Carthami* and 9 grams of *Radix Angelicae Sinensis*. In case of invasion of ying system by heat marked by coma, delirium, deep-red tongue, absence of nasal discharge and tears, the above prescription and *Decoction for clearing away heat in ying system* should include *Radix Curcumae* and *Rhizoma Acori Graminei* which are to be decocted for oral administration. Simultaneously, *Purple Snowy Powder* should be taken after being infused in the finished decoction of the above ingredients.

4. Stagnation of Phlegm-dampness in the Lung

Main Symptoms and Signs: Cough, shortness of breath, phlegm-dyspnea, rale in the throat, yellowish face and pale lips, sometimes cold and heat, red tongue with greasy fur, and smooth pulse.

Therapeutic Principles: Drying the dampness evil, eliminating phlegm, and relieving the cough and asthma.

Recipe: *Xiaoqinglong tang (Minor decoction of green dragon) and Erchen tang (Two old drugs decoction)*, modified.

Herba Ephedrae 6 g
Ramulus Cinnamomi 3 g
Semen Armeniacae Amarum 3 g
Rhizoma Pinelliae 9 g
Pericarpium Citri Reticulatae 6 g
Semen Lepidii seu Descurainiae 6 g
Herba Asari 1.5 g
Fructus Schisandrae 4.5 g
Radix Glycyrrhizae 3 g

Decoct the above ingredients in a right amount of water for oral administration.

5. Deficiency of Healthy Energy due to Remaining Pathogens

It is commonly seen during the later stage of the disease. The healthy energy is deficient while the pathogenic factor is not all removed.

1) **Lung - heat due to Yin - deficiency**

Main Symptoms and Signs: Low fever, night sweat, flushed face, unproductive cough, dry mouth with red lips, red and dry tongue without fur coating, and fine and rapid pulse.

Therapeutic Principles: Nourishing yin and clearing away lung - heat.

Recipe: *Shashen Maidong tang* (*Decoction of Adenophorae Strictae and Ophiopogonis*), modified.

Radix Adenophorae Strictae	12 g
Radix Ophiopogonis	9 g
Rhizoma Polygonati Odorali	9 g
Cortex Mori Radicis	12 g
Cortex Lycii Radicis	12 g
Radix Trichosanthis	9 g
Semen Dolichoris	9 g
Semen Armeniacae	6 g
Radix Glycyrrhizae	3 g

Decoct the above ingredients in a right amount of water for oral administration.

Modification: If cough is severe, *Folium Eriobotryae* 9 g, *Radix Stemanae* 9 g, and *Bulbus Fritillariae Cirrhosae* 6 g should be added to relieve cough and resolve phlegm; if associated with poor appetite, *Fructus Crutaegi* 9 g and *Fructus Hordei Germinatus* 9 g, added to relieve dyspepsia and promote appetite.

2) **Qi - deficiency of Lung and Spleen**

Main Symptoms and Signs: Irregular low fever, weak cough with low sound and thin sputum, pale complexion, listlessness, spontaneous perspiration, poor appetite, loose stools, pale tongue with whitish and smooth fur, and fine and faint pulse.

Therapeutic Principles: Benefiting the qi and invigorating the spleen.

Recipe: *Renshen wuweizi tang* (*Decoction of Codonopsis Pilosula and Schisandra*), modified.

Radix Lodonopsis Pilosulae	12 g
Radix Astragali seu Hedysari	12 g
Rhizoma Atractylodis Macrocephalae Praeparatae	9 g
Poria	9 g
Fructus Schisandrae	6 g
Rhizoma Pinelliae	9 g
Radix Glycyrrhizae Praeparatae	3 g

Decoct the above ingredients in a right amount of water for oral administration.

Modification: If there is productive cough, *Radix Asteris* 9 g, *Pericarpium Citri Reticulatae* 6 g and *Arisaema cum Bile* 9 g should be added to relieve cough and resolve phlegm; for deficiency of ying and wei, profuse sweating and weakened breathing, *Ramulus Cinnamomi* 6 g, *Concha Astreae* 15 g and *Os Draconis* 15 g are applicable to regulate ying and wei and, stop excessive perspiration, and strengthen yang – energy.

6. Special Syndromes

1) Liver – wind Stirring

Main Symptoms and Signs: High fever, mental cloudiness, restlessness, irritability, delirium, convulsion, staring upward, neck rigidity, a deep – red tongue with yellow and coarse coating, and a wiry and rapid pulse.

this syndrome is due to direct invasion of the heart and liver by excessive heat toxins. Invasion of the heart causes mental cloudiness and delirium. Heat – toxins stir liver wind with the ensuing symptoms of convulsion. A deep – red tongue with yellow and coarse coating, and a wiry and rapid pulse are both signs of excess of heat – toxins.

Therapeutic Principles: Clearing heat in the heart, cooling the liver, calming the wind and promoting mental resuscitation.

Recipe: *Lingjiao gouteng tang* (*Decoction of Cornu Antolopis and Ramulus Uncariae cum Uncis*)

Cornu Antolopis	1 g
Ramulus Uncariae cum Uncis	10 g
Rhizoma Rehmanniae	10 g
Radix Paeoniae Alba	10 g
Bulbus Fritillariae Cirrhosae	5 g
Cortex Mori Radicis	10 g
Rhizoma Acori Graminei	5 g

Cornu Antolopis is ground into powder and dissolved in water and taken separately.

This prescription clears heat in the heart, promotes mental resuscitation, cools the liver and calms wind. *Cornu Antolopis* and *Ramulus Uncariae cum Uncis* soothe the liver and calm wind. *Rhizoma Rehmanniae* cools blood. *Radix Paeoniae Alba* nourishes the liver. *Bulbus Fritillariae Cirrhosae* and *Cortex Mori Radicis* clear heat in the lung and resolve phlegm. *Rhizoma Acori Graminei* promotes mental resuscitation.

2) **Exhaustion of Heart - yang**

Main Symptoms and Signs: Pale complexion, restlessness, cyanosis of lips and nails, cold limbs, sweating, rapid enlargement of the liver, a dark - purplish or pale tongue, and a feeble, thready and rapid pulse.

This syndrome is due to serious blockage of lung - qi, resulting in stagnation of qi and blood. The retarded circulation of heart blood causes cyanosis. Since the liver stores blood, stagnation of blood enlarges the liver rapidly. Insufficient nourishment for the heart weakens heart - qi, causing pale complexion and cold limbs. In the case of exhaustion of heart - yang, the heart is unable to dominate blood vessels, resulting in a feeble, thready and rapid pulse or even a fading pulse.

Therapeutic Principles: To recapture yang and rescue the collapsing state.

Recipe: *Shenfu longmu jiuni tang*

Radix Ginseng	10 g
Radix Aconiti Praeparata	10 g
Radix Glycyrrhizae Praeparata	5 g
Radix Paeoniae Alba	10 g
Os Draconis	20 g
Concha Ostreae	20 g

This prescription benefits qi, checks discharge, recaptures yang and rescues the collapsing state. *Radix Ginseng* benefits qi and tonifies the heart. *Radix Aconiti Praeparata* warms yang and rescues the collapsing state. *Radix Paeoniae Alba* and *Radix Glycyrrhizae Praeparata* protect yin. *Os Draconis* and *Concha Ostreae* suppress yang.

OTHER THERAPIES

1. Simple Recipe and Proved Prescription

1) *Herba Houttuyniae Injection* can be used intramuscularly, one for each time, one or twice daily or 5 - 10 ml drug solution, put into 5 - 10% *glucos solution* (200 ml) given by intravenous drip, or a mixture of physiological *saline solution* 10 ml and drug solution 10 ml is given through aerosol inhalation. This is applicable to common pneumonia of children.

2) *Feiyan Heji*. It is composed of:

Semen Ginkgo	9 g
Indigo Naturalis	3 g
Cortex Lycii Radicis	9 g
Ramulus Uncariae cum Uncis	9 g

Herba Plantaginis 9 g
Pericarpium Citri Reticulatae 9 g

Decoct the above ingredients in a right amount of water for oral administration.

3) *Bingduxing Feiyan Heji*. It is composed of:

Folium Isatidis 15 g
Radix Isatidis 15 g
Herba Plantaginis 9 g
Radix Bupleuri 9 g
Bombyx Batryticatus 9 g

Decoct the above ingredients in a right amount of water for oral administration.

4) *Chuanke San*

Rhizoma Pinelliae and *Fructus Schisandrae*, 3 portions of each, and *Herba Asari* and *Rhizoma Zingiberis*, one portion of each, all together are made into powder and taken after being infused, 2 g each time, 2 – 3 times daily or decocted in proper amount of water over a soft fire 2 – 3 minutes, for one drink after removing the dregs.

2. External Application

Semen Sinapis Ablae 30 g and *flour* 30 g are mixed with some water, wrapped with gauze, which can be applied to the back area of a patient, once daily for 15 minutes till the skin turns red, which continues for three days. This method has a significant effect for the patient with persisting lung rales.

3. Acupuncture Treatment

1) Excess Syndromes

Therapeutic Principles: To disperse wind – cold for cold syndrome, and to clear heat and resolve phlegm or to clear heat and promote the lung's function in dispersing for heat syndromes. Points from the *Urinary Bladder* and *Lung Meridians* are mainly selected and needled with reducing method.

Prescription: Fengmen(**BL**12), Feishu(**BL**13), Chize(**LU**5), Lieque(**LU**7), Fenglong (**ST**40)

Explanation: Fengmen(**BL**12) eliminates wind. Feishu(**BL**13) promotes the lung's function in dispersing. Chize(**LU**5), the son point of the *Lung Meridian*, is given the reducing method.

Prescription: Shuigou(**DU**26), Baihui(**DU**20), the 12 Jing – Well Points, Shenmen (**HT**7), Dazhui(**DU**14), Quchi(**LI**11).

Points according to symptoms and signs:

Convulsion: Shousanli(**LI**10), Waiguan(**SJ**5), Yanglingquan(**GB**34), Taichong(**LR**3) through to Yongquan(**KI**1).

Staring upward: Cuanzhu(**BL**2), Jingming(**BL**1).

Neck rigidity: Fengfu(DU16), Tianzhu(BL10).

Expalnation: Dazhui(DU14)and Quchi(LI11) clear heat. Shenmen(HT7) clears heat in the heart and calms the mind. Shuigou(DU26), Baihui(DU20) and the 12 Jing – Well Points clear heat, refresh the brain and promote mental resuscitation.

2) **Exhaustion of Heart – yang**

Therapeutic Principles: To recapture yang and rescue the collapsing state. Needling with the reinforcing method is combined with moxibustion.

Prescription: Baihui(DU20), Yintang(EX – HN3), Shenque(RN8) with salt, Guanyuan (RN4), Zusanli(ST36).

Explanation: Baihui(DU20) and Yintang(EX – HN3) refresh the brain. Zusanli(ST36) benefits qi. Shenque(RN8) and Guanyuan(RN4) recapture yang and rescue the collapsing state.

4. **Cupping**

Cupping, for pneumonia of the late stage with persistent rale, is applied to the lower part of the scapula on both sides generally, or just on the side where rale is obviously localized. Local ecchymoses may occur after cupping, but blisters are not to be caused. The cup is attached to the skin for 5 – 10 minutes each time. Treatment is given once a day, five sessions consisted of one course.

PREVENTION AND NURSING

1. Prevention

1) It is advisable for the patient to do more physical exercise so as to build up health and prevent cold.

2) Outdoor activities are recomended and fresh air in the living room is also helpful. Besides, attention should be paid to the changing of clothes according to different weather.

3) Active measures should be taken to prevent malnutrition, rickets, measles, whooping cough and cold, etc..

2. **Nursing**

1) The patient's room must be kept quiet with flowing air, proper temperature and humidity.

2) If there is much sputum, the body position of the patient should be frequently changed so that the sputum can be drawn out or eliminated by means of ligh pats on the back. Oxygen is indicated for patients who are cyanotic and dyspneic.

3) The patient should keep a diet of light and easily digested food, avoiding greasy

food, meat or fish lest sputum and heat should be produced.

4) Special attention should be paid to the conditions of severe patients.

Chapter Twelve
Lobar Pneumonia

Pneumococcal pneumonia, an inflammatory process in the lung parenchyma, is an acute bacterial infection of the lungs. It is caused by *pneumococcus* and characterized clinically by an abrupt onset with rigor, fever, chest pain, cough and blood sputum.

Pneumococcal pneumonia may occur at any season, but is most common during winter and early spring when viral respiratory infections are most prevalent.

The *pneumococcus* accounts for 60 – 80% of community – acquired bacterial pneumonia. These bacteria frequently are in the normal flora of the respiratory tract. The development of pneumonia therefore usually is attributed to the impairment of natural resistance. Conditions leading to aspiration of secretions include suppression of the cough, or epiglottic reflex impairment of upward migration of mucous sheets (propelled by cilia) and impairment of alveolar phagocyte function. Among conditions that predispose to pneumonia are viral respiratory diseases, malnutrition, exposure to cold, noxious gases, alcohol intoxication, depression of cerebral functions by drugs and cardiac failure. Pulmonary consolidation may be in one or more lobes or may be patchy in distribution.

In traditional Chinese medicine, this disorder is termed *seasonal disease*, *ke sou*, but the symptoms are equal to those of wind and warm symptom complex and winter fever or suppurative infections of the lungs and are thought to belong to acute febrile disease caused by pathogenic wind and warm factors in spring and winter orr caused by different warm pathogenic factors in different seasons.

ETIOLOGY AND PATHOGENESIS

Invasion of the lung by pathogenic wind – heat through mouth and nose leads to accumulation of phlegm – heat and dysfunction of the lung in purification and dispersion, giving rise to cough and chest pain.

Irregular daily life or sudden change of the weather makes the superficial defensive qi fail to adjust its defending function; overstrain impairs the function of the spleen and kidney; affection of the six exopathogens or seasonal pathogens leads to stagnation of qi and lung – heat, which heats the fluid into phlegm; combination of phlegm and heat impairs pulmonary vessels. The above factors get together to form the cause of this disease. When the vital qi is strong and the pathogens have been driven away, the phlegm – heat will accordingly vanish. If the fever is high, the vital qi will be exhausted.

MAIN SYMPTOMS AND SIGNS

Victims of pneumococcal pneumonia are often found seriously ill. The onset is usually sudden with shaking chills, "stabbing" chest pain (exaggerated by respiration but sometimes referred to the shoulder, abdomen or flank), high fever, cough and "rusty" sputum and occasionally vomiting.

The patient appears severely ill with marked tachypnea (30 – 40% min) but no orthopnea. Respirations are grunting and the patient often lies on the affected side in an attempt to splint the chest. Herpes simplex facial lesions are often present.

Initially, chest excursion is diminished on the involved side. Breath sounds are suppressed and fine inspiratory rales are heard. Later, the classic signs (absent breath sound, dullness, etc.) of consolidation appear. A pleural friction rub or abodminal distention amy be present. During resolution of the pneumonia, the signs of consolidation are replaced by rales. Physical findings are often inconclusive and repeated x – ray examination is helpful. Constant features of the disease are fever and toxemia with the temperature usually ranging between 103 and 106 F. During the febrile period complaints of malaise, anorexia, weakness, myalgia and general prostration are extremely common.

MAIN POINTS OF DIAGNOSIS

1. This disease is usually caused by pathogenic wind (cold, heat and pestilential factors), overfatigue, mental injury or asthenia after illness.

2. It is characterized by chillness, fever, cough, chest pain, and yellow or rusty sputum.

3. Dry or wet rale can be heard on auscultation and dull resonance of the lung on percussion. The X – ray examination of the patient at the stage consolidation shows patchy shadow with an even increase in density.

4. With the blood test, it could be found that the total white blood cells is over 10, 000/mm^3, the value of neutrophilic granulocytes is over 70% with the nucleus shifting to the left.

5. *Pneumococci* are present in the sputum and often in the blood.

6. Newly – contracted acute febrile diseases or seasonal diseases including the wind and warm symptom complex and winter fever or suppurative infections of the lungs in traditional Chinese medicine.

7. In severe cases, there might appear semiconsciousness or even coma accompanied by a fall of blood pressure, cold sweating and pallor, which indicate peripheral circulatory

failure.

DIFFERENTIATION AND TREATMENT OF COMMON SYNDROMES

1. Dysfunction of the lung in dispersing due to invasion by pathogenic warm.

Main Symptoms and Signs: Chillness, fever (with sudden rise of body temperature up to over 38℃), headache, general ache, chest pain, bad cough with sticky expectoration, thin and white tongue coating or thin, yellow coating with less fluid, and superficial and rapid pulse.

Therapeutic Principles: Clearing heat, dispelling wind, dispersing the lung and arresting cough.

Recipe: *Yinqiao san* (*Powder of Lonicerae and Forsythiae*), modified.

Flos Lonicerae	30 g
Fructus Forsythiae	12 g
Herba Houttuyniae	30 g
Herba Menthae	9 g
Semen Armeniacae	9 g
Radix Platycodi	9 g
Rhizoma Phragmitis	30 g
Herba Lophatheri	3 g
Fructus Arctii	12 g
Fructus Trichosanthis	24 g
Indigo Naturalis	6 g
Radix Glycyrrhizae	6 g

Decoct the above ingredients in a right amount of water for oral administration.

Modification: In case of high fever, add *Gypsum Fibrosum* 30–45 g.

In case of high fever with coma, add 1.5 g of *Lingyang fen* (*powder of Cornu Antelopis*) to be taken following its infusion.

2. Preponderance of Heat in the Lung and Stomach Leading to Intense Heat in the Ying and Blood System

Main Symptoms and Signs: High fever (over 39℃), severe cough, coarse breathing, burning pain in the chest, massive expectoration of rusty or blood-stained purulent sputum, polyhidrosis, thirst, red face, constipation, yellow and dry tongue coating, and full or full and rapid pulse.

Therapeutic Principles: Clearing away heat from the lung and stomach, and cooling toxic heat from the blood system.

Recipe: *Yinqiao baihu tang*, modified.

Flos Lonicerae	30 g
Fructus Forsythiae	12 g
Folium Isatidis	30 g
Herba Patriniae	30 g
Herba Houttuyniae	30 g
Rhizoma Anemarrhenae	12 g
Gypsum Fibrosum	45 g
Cortex Mori Radicis	30 g
Radix Rehmanniae	30 g
Semen Persicae	15 g
Semen Coicis	30 g

Decoct the above ingredients in a right amount of water twice to obtain 300 ml of decoction to be taken half in the morning and half in the evening while it is warm.

Modification: In case of severe cough with chest pain, add *Bulbus Fritillariae Thunbergii* 12 g, *Radix Curcumae* 12 g and *Pericarpium Trichosanthis* 15 g.

In case of constipation with absence of bowel movement for days, add *Rhizoma et Radix Rhei* 12 g, *Natrii Sulfas* 9 – 12 g (to be taken following its infusion) and *Fructus Trichosanthis* 30 g.

Impairment of Yin of the Lung and Stomach

Main Symptoms and Signs: Gradual fall of high fever, or persistent low – grade fever, decrease of expectoration of blood – stained sputum, mental restlessness, thirst, red tongue with little coating, and thready and rapid pulse.

Therapeutic Principles: Nourishing yin of the stomach, moistening the lung and clearing away the heat from the lung.

Recipe: *Zhuye shigao tang* and *Yangyin qingfei tang*

Gypsum Fibrosum	30 g
Radix Ophiopogonis	30 g
Radix Pseudostellariae	30 g
Herba Lophatheri	3 g
Cortex Moutan Radicis	9 g
Radix Rehmanniae	15 g
Radix Scrophulariae	15 g
Radix Paeoniae Alba	12 g

Bulbus Fritillariae Cirrhosae 12 g

Decoct the above ingredients in a right amount of water twice to obtain 300 ml of decoction to be taken half in the morning and half in the evening while it is warm.

Modification: In case of constipation, add *Rhizoma et Radix Rhei* 9 g and *Fructus Cannabis* 30 g.

4. **Pathogens Invading the Lung**

Main Symptoms and Signs: Fever, aversion to cold, difficulty in coughing, fullness and oppressed feeling in the chest, or vague pain in the chest, little white sticky sputum, no or little sweat, thirst, or headache, general discomfort, sore throat, stuffy nose, reddened tongue tip and margin, thin whitish or thin yellowish tongue coating, and floating rapid pulse.

Therapeutic Principles: Relieving exterior syndrome with drugs pungent in flavor and cool in nature, facilitating the flow of the lung-qi.

Recipe: *Modified yinqiao san* (*Powder of Lonicera and forsythia*) and *Sangju yin* (*Decoction of Mulberry leaf and Chrysanthemum*)

Flos Lonicerae	30 g
Rhizoma Phragmitis	30 g
Fructus Forsythiae	15 g
Folium Mori	9 g
Semen Armenicae Amarum	9 g
Radix Platycodi	9 g
Radix Peucedani	9 g
Bulbus Fritillariae Thunbergii	9 g
Fructus Arctii	9 g
Radix Glycyrrhizae	3 g

Decoct the above ingredients in a right amount of water for oral administration.

Modification: For severe chills and anhidrosis, the drugs added are *Herba Ephedrae* 9 g, *Folium Perillae* 9 g.

For high fever, profuse sweat and thirst, the drugs added are *Gypsum Fibrosum* 30 g, *Rhizoma Anemarrhenae* 12 g.

For headache and general aching, the drugs added are *Flos Chrysanthemi* 9 g, *Fructus Viticis* 9 g and *Radix Puerariae* 15 g.

Chinese Patent Medicine: *Fangfeng tongsheng wan* (*Miraculous pill of Ledebouriella*)

Indications: Aversion to cold, high fever, constipation and deep-colored urine in the early stage of pneumonia.

Administration: Taken orally, 6 g each time, twice daily.

Caution: It should be cautiously used for pregnant women.

Phlegm – heat Retained in the Lung

Main Symptoms and Signs: Persistent high fever, frequent cough, yellow sticky or rusty or bloody sputum which is in moderate amount, raucous breathing, falring of nares, aggravated chest pain, restlessness, thirst with desire for more drinking, flushed face, reddened tongue with yellowish dry coating, and full slippery pulse.

Therapeutic Principles: Clearing away heat in the lung to relieve asthma, arresting cough and resolving phlegm.

Recipe:

Flos Lonicerae	30 g
Herba Taraxaci	30 g
Flos Chrysanthemi Indici	15 g
Herba Violae	15 g
Fructus Trichosanthis	15 g
Radix Semiaquilegiae	15 g
Rhizoma Coptidis	9 g
Rhizoma Pinelliae	9 g
Semen Benincasae	15 g
Semen Armenicae Amarum	9 g
Bulbus Fritillariae Thunbergii	9 g
Semen Lepidii seu Descurainiae	15 g

Decoct the above ingredients in a right amount of water for oral administration.

Modification: In case of bloody sputum, the drugs added are *Herba Cirsii* 30 g, *Rhizoma Imperatae* 30 g and *Nodus Nelumbinis Rhizomatis* 30 g.

In case of severe cough and dyspnea, the drugs added are *Herba Ephedrae Praeparata* 9 g, *Fructus Perillae* 9 g.

In case of stabbing pain in the chest and cyanotic lips, the drugs added are *Semen Persicae* 9 g, *Radix Paeoniae Rubra* 15 g and *Radix Salviae Miltiorrhizae* 15 g.

Chinese Patent Medicine

Lingyang qingfei wan (*Antelope's horn pill for removing heat from the lung*)

Indications: High fever, yellow sputum, shortness of breath, chest pain, dark urine and dry stools.

Administration: Taken orally, 6 g each time, 3 times daily.

Used cautiously for pregnant women.

6. Invasion of Heat into the Heart – ying

Main Symptoms and Signs: High fever which is severe in the night, cough, shortness of breath, rale in the throat, yellowish thick or bloody sputum, chest pain, thirst without desire for drinking, even unconsciousness, dysphoria, delirium, involuntary movement of the hands and feet, dark reddened dry tongue with dry and yellow coating, and deep thready rapid pulse.

Therapeutic Principles: Clearing up the ying－system, detoxicating, inducing resuscitation and calming the endopathic wind.

Recipe:

Cornu Rhinocerotis	1.5 g
Flos Lonicerae	30 g
Fructus Forsythiae	15 g
Radix Rehmanniae	12 g
Radix Scrophulariae	12 g
Radix Ophiopogonis	12 g
Radix Salviae Miltiorrhizae	12 g
Herba Lophatheri	9 g
Rhizoma Coptidis	9 g
Concretio Silicea Bambusae	9 g
Arisaema cum Bile	9 g

Decoct the above ingredients in a right amount of water for oral administration.

Modification: If there is abundant heat in the ying－blood system and blood spots on the skin, the drugs added are *Folium Isatidis* 30 g, *Radix Arnebiae seu Lithospermi* 15 g, and *Radix Paeoniae Rubra* 15 g.

If there is convulsion due to excessive endopathogenic wind, the drugs added are *Cornu Saigae Tataricae* 3 g (in the form of powder taken after being infused in water), *Scorpio* in the form of powder 3 g (taken after being infused in water).

If there is rale in the throat, dyspnea, and phlegm－accumulation due to stagnancy of the lung－qi, the drugs added are *Calculus Macacae* 0.6 g, *Succus Bambosae* 20 ml (The above two drugs are taken after being infused in water).

If there is coma and delirium, the drugs added are *Radix Curcumae* 12 g, *Rhizoma Acori Tatarinowii* 12 g.

Chinese Patent Medicine: *Wanshi niuhuang qingxin wan* (*Wan's bezoar sedative bolus*)

Indications: High fever and convulsion.

Administration: Taken orally, 3 g each time, 2－3 times daily.

7. Type of Exhausting Vital－qi

Main Symptoms and Signs: Sudden drop of the body temperature, hyperhidrosis of the head, cold limbs, weak breathing, feeble cough, noise like snore in the throat, cyanosis of the lips and nails, unconsciousness, or dysphoria, pale complexion, or flushing of the zygomatic region, dry mouth, dark red tongue with little dry coating, and feeble thready pulse.

Therapeutic Principles: Supplementing qi to nourish yin, recuperating depleted yang to hold back the exhaustion of vital-qi.

Recipe:

Radix Ginseng	3-6 g
Radix Ophiopogonis	15 g
Fructus Schisandrae	6 g
Radix Aconiti Lateralis Praeparata	6-9 g
Os Draconis Fossilia	15 g
Concha Ostreae	15 g

Decoct the above ingredients in a right amount of water for oral administration.

Modification: If the main symptom is yin depletion, the drugs added are *Radix Glehniae* 12 g and *Fructus Corni* 12 g.

If the main symptom is yang exhaustion, the drugs added are *Rhizoma Zingiberis* 9 g and *Cortex Cinnamomi* 6 g.

8. Deteriorated Syndromes

1) Excessive Heat in the Lung and Stomach Leading to Impairment of both Qi and Yin

Main Symptoms and Signs: High fever, cough, chest pain, coarse breathing, expectoration of bloody or rusty sputum, polyhidrosis, thirst, red tongue with yellow and dry coating hollow and rapid pulse.

Therapeutic Principles: Clearing away pathogenic heat from the lung and stomach, tonifying qi and nourishing yin.

Recipe:

Flos Lonicerae	30 g
Fructus Forsythiae	15 g
Herba houttuyniae	30 g
Gypsum Fibrosum	45 g
Rhizoma Anemarrhenae	12 g
Radix Pannacis Quinquefolii	15 g
Radix Pseudostellariae	30 g
Radix Ophiopogonis	30 g
Cortex Mori	15 g

Decoct the above ingredients in a right amount of water twice to obtain 300 ml of decoction to be taken half in the morning and half in the evening while it is warm.

2) **Collapse due to Exhaustion of Yang**

Main Symptoms and Signs: Sudden drop of high fever (down to below 36℃), profuse cold sweating, pallor, sudden fall of blood pressure (with systolic pressure below 80 mmHg), oliguria, fading or rapid and faint pulse.

Therapeutic Principles: Restoring yang and rescuing the patient from the collapse.

Recipe 1:

Radix Ginseng 30 g

Decoct the above ingredients in a right amount of water twice to obtain 200 ml of decoction. Take it while it is warm.

Recipe 2:

Radix Ginseng 15 g
Radix Aconiti Praeparata 30 g
Fructus Evodiae 15 g
Semen Schisandrae 9 g

Decoct the above ingredients in a right amount of water twice to obtain 200 ml of decoction. Take it while it is warm.

Recipe 3:

Radix Ginseng 12 g
Radix Ophiopogonis 24 g
Fructus Schisandrae 9 g
Radix Aconiti Praeparata 15 g
Rhizoma Zingiberis 12 g
Radix Glycyrrhizae Praeparata 6 g

Decoct the above ingredients in a right amount of water twice to obtain 200 ml of decoction. Take it while it is warm.

Besides, add 10 ml of *Shen Fu Injection* or *Sheng Mai Injection* to 500 ml of 10% *glucose solution* for intravenous drip, once to twice daily.

Pneumococcal pneumonia is classified into three types by other researchers.

1. **The Wei Phase of the Lung**

Main Symptoms and Signs: The clinical features at early stages are chills and fever, thirst, perspiration, cough and headache with thin white or yellowish coating of the tongue and superficial and rapid pulse.

Therapeutic Principles: To treat external symptom complex by using drugs with cold property.

Recipe:

Honeysuckle flower	15 – 30 g
Weeping forsythia	15 – 30 g
Bamboo leaves	10 g
Schizonepeta tenuifolia	12 g
Achene of great burdock	10 g
Peppermint	10 g
Common reed rhizome	30 g
Root of balloonflower	12 g
Root of figwort	15 – 30 g
Tuber of dwarf lilyturf	18 g
Fresh or dried root of rehmannia	18 g
Gypsum	30 – 60 g
Licorice root	6 g

Decoct the above ingredients in a right amount of water twice to obtain 300 ml of decoction to be taken half in the morning and half in the evening while it is warm.

2. **Excess Heat**

Main Symptoms and Signs: High fever, anxiety, profuse sweating, thirst, flushed face, deep colored urine, constipation, cough and yellowish and dry coating of the tongue, and full and large pulse.

Therapeutic Principles: Purifying the qi with pungent and cold drugs.

Recipe:

Chinese ephedra	10 g
Apricot kernel	12 g
Gypsum	30 – 60 g
Root – bark of white mulberry	30 g
Root of purple – flowered peucedanum	15 g
Tatarian aster	24 g
Common coltsfoot flower	10 g
Tendril – leaved fritillary bulb	10 g
Cordate houttuynia	30 – 60 g
Skullcap root	10 g

Decoct the above ingredients in a right amount of water twice to obtain 300 ml of decoction to be taken half in the morning and half in the evening while it is warm.

3. **Suppurative Infections of the Lungs**

Main Symptoms and Signs: Suppuration, cough, foul – smelling of the sputum. He may or may not have high fever. Yellow coating of the tongue and large full pulse are present.

Therapeutic Principles: Dissipating heat and detoxifying the lung.

Recipe:

Common reed rhizome	30 g
Cordate houttuynia	30 – 60 g
Skullcap root	10 g
Root – bark of white mulbery	30 g
Apricot kernel	12 g
Root of purple – flowered peucedanum	15 g
Root of balloonflower	12 – 15 g
Chinese goldthread rhizome	6 – 10 g
Dandelio	30 g
Herba patrinia	30 g
Peach kernel	12 g

PREVENTION

Take an active part in physical training regularly and try the best to prevent cold and bronchitis.

Chapter Thirteen
Obstructive Emphysema

Obstructive emphysema in traditional Chinese medicine is included in the category of *lung distention*, which is clinically characterized by asthma and distending sensation in the chest. Intermittent attack of chronic bronchitis, bronchial asthma, extensive bronchiectasis and chronic fibro – cavitative pulmonary tuberculosis leads to obstruction of bronchiole, which causes over – filing of the termina lends of bronchiole resulting in elasticity decline of lung tissue and volume increase of the lung; thus bringing about this disease.

ETIOLOGY AND PATHOGENESIS

Protracted and improperly – treated chronic disorders of the pulmonary system such as codl, cough, dyspnea, asthma, pulmonary abscess and lung atrophy cause deficiency of all the lung, spleen and kidney, and disturbance of qi, blood and body fluids in transportation and distribution, which brings about retention of phlegm, stasis of blood, block of the respiratory tract, and, in turn, inflation of the lung – qi failing to astringe and descend, exhaustion of the qi of the lower – jiao, and failure of the kidney to hold inspiration. Repeated attack of the six exopathogens at this time will evoke the acute onset of cough, dyspnea, asthma, etc..

DIFFERENTIATION AND TREATMENT OF COMMON SYNDROMES

1. Exterior Syndrome of Excess Type

1) Exterior Cold and Interior Heat

Main Symptoms and Signs: Severe chills, mild fever, stuffy nose with watery discharge, anhidrosis, asthma with hoarse breathing, yellow sticky thick sputum, reddened tongue with yellowish coating, and slippery rapid pulse.

Therapeutic Principles: Relieving exterior syndrome and clearing away internal heat.

Recipe:

Herba Ephedrae Praeparata 9 g
Ramulus Cinnamomi 9 g
Semen Armeniacae Amarum 9 g
Bulbus Fritillariae Thunbergii 9 g

Fructus Trichosanthis 15 g
Gypsum Fibrosum 30 g
Radix Glycyrrhizae 4.5 g

Decoct the above ingredients in a right amount of water for oral administration.

Modification: If external－cold symptoms are severe, the drugs added are *Folium Perillae* 9 g, *Rhizoma seu Radix Notopterygii* 9 g.

If yellow sputum is in large amount, sticky and difficult to expectorate, the drugs added are *Semen Benincasae* 30 g, *Os Costaziae* 30 g, *Semen Coicis* 30 g.

If cough and asthma are severe, the drugs added are *Radix Stemonae* 12 g, *Fructus Perillae* 12 g, *Cortex Mori* 12 g.

Chinese Patent Medicine: *Qingwen jiedu wan* (*Antipyretic and antitoxic pill*)

Taken orally, 9 g each time, 3 times daily.

2) **Cold－phlegm Accumulated in the Lung**

Main Symptoms and Signs: Frequent expectoration of white frothy sputum, chills, cold limbs, protracted cough and asthma which are evoked whenever cold is affected, whitish slippery tongue coating, and taut slippery slow pulse.

Therapeutic Principles: Warming and resolving cold－phlegm.

Recipe:

Cortex Magnoliae Officinalis 9 g
Herba Ephedrae Praeparata 9 g
Semen Armeniacae Amarum 9 g
Rhizoma Pinelliae 9 g
Rhizoma Zingiberis 9 g
Fructus Schisandrae 6 g
Herba Asari 3 g

Decoct the above ingredients in a right amount of water for oral administration.

Modification: In case of profuse sputum, the drug added is *Poria* 30 g.

In case of aversion to cold, fever and absence of sweat, the drugs added are *Ramulus Cinnamomi* 9 g, *Herba Schizonepetae* 9 g.

In case of cough and asthma which make one lying down impossible, the drugs added are *Fructus Perillae* 12 g, *Radix Asteris* 9 g and *Flos Farfarae* 9 g.

In case of chills and cold limbs, the drug added is *Radix Aconiti Lateralis Praeparata* 6 g.

Chinese Patent Medicine: *Mahuang zhisou wan* (*Ephedra pill for arresting cough*)

Taken orally, 6 g each time, twice to 3 times daily.

3) **Phlegm – heat Retained in the Lung**

Main Symptoms and Signs: White sticky or yellow thick profuse sputum, distending full and oppressed sensation in the chest, cough, asthma, or fever, flushed face, thirst, dark urine, dry stools, reddened tongue with yellow thick coating, and full slippery pulse.

Therapeutic Principles: Clearing away the lung – heat, resolving phlegm, checking upward adverse flow of qi and relieving asthma.

Recipe:

Gypsum Fibrosum	30 g
Semen Trichosanthis	24 g
Radix Scutellariae	9 g
Semen Armeniacae Amarum	9 g
Pericarpium Citri Reticulatae	9 g
Rhizoma Pinelliae	9 g
Poria	9 g
Arisaema cum Bile	9 g
Fructus Aurantii Immaturus	9 g
Radix et Rhizoma Rhei	4.5 g

Decoct the above ingredients in a right amount of water for oral administration.

Modification: In case of difficulty in expectoration, the drugs added are *Concha Meretricis seu Cyclinae* (in the form of powder) 15 g, *Os Costaziae* 15 g, *Natrii Sulfas Exsiccatus* 9 g.

In case of asthma with rale in the throat and incapability of lying flat when sleeping, the drugs added are *Lumbricus* 12 g, *Cortex Magnoliae Officinalis* 9 g.

In case of body – fluid impaired by phlegm – heat and dry mouth and throat, the drugs added are *Radix Trichosanthis* 12 g, *Rhizoma Anemarrhenae* 12 g and *Rhizoma Phragmitis* 24 g.

Chinese Patent Medicine

1. *Qingfei yihuo wan* (*Pill for clearing away heat in the lung and controlling fire*)

Administration: Taken orally, 6 g each time, 2 times daily.

Caution: Contraindicated for pregnant women.

2. *Houzao san* (*Monkey bezoar powder*)

Indications: Those with blocked orifices due to phlegm – heat, unconsciousness and stridor.

Administration: Taken orally, 0.3 – 0.6 g each time, once or twice daily.

4) **Blood Retained in the Lung**

Main Symptoms and Signs: Asthma, shortness of breath, flaring of nares, cyanosis of face, distending and oppressed sensation and dull pain in the chest, dark red tongue with ecchymoses, sublingual varices, thin white tongue coating, and sunken choppy pulse.

Therapeutic Principles: Activating blood – flow to remove blood stasis

Recipe:

Radix Rehmanniae	12 g
Radix Paeoniae Rubra	12 g
Radix Angelicae Sinensis	12 g
Semen Persicae	9 g
Flos Carthami	9 g
Rhizoma Chuanxiong	9 g

Decoct the above ingredients in a right amount of water for oral administration.

Modification: In case of fever, flushed face, restlessness, and thirst, the drugs added are *Flos Lonicerae* 24 g, *Herba Houttuyniae* 24 g, *Fructus Forsythiae* 12 g.

In case of accumulation of profuse phlegm, the drugs added are *Exocarpium Citri Reticulatae* 9 g, *Rhizoma Pineliae* 9 g, *Radix Peucedani* 9 g, *Poria* 12 g and *Semen Trichosanthis* 12 g.

In case of shortness of breath and palpitation which are aggravated when moving, the drugs added are *Radix Astragali* 30 g, *Radix Codonopsis* 30 g.

In case of remarkable cough and asthma, the drugs added are *Semen Armeniacae Amarum* 9 g, *Bulbus Fritillariae Cirrhosae* 9 g, *Radix Asteris* 12 g and *Flos Farfarae* 12 g.

2. Interior Syndrome of Deficiency Type

1) Qi – deficiency of the Lung and Kidney

Main Symptoms and Signs: Shortness of breath with the mouth opened and the shoulders shrugged when the patient is still, cough with low noise, chills, spontaneous sweating, being susceptible to cold, etc..

Therapeutic Principles: Tonifying the lung and nourishing the kidney.

Recipe:

Radix Ginseng	(taken after being stewed in water) 3 g
Radix Astragali	30 g
Cortex Cinnamomi	1.5 g
Cobblestone	1.5 g
Fructus Schisandrae	6 g
Radix Glycyrrhizae Praeparata	6 g

Decoct the above ingredients in a right amount of water for oral administration.

Modification: For profuse sweating, the drugs added are

Fructus Tritici Levis	30 g
Concha Ostreae	30 g
Radix Ephedrae	9 g

Chinese Patent Medicine: *Lingzhi pian* (*Lucid Ganoderma Tablet*)

Taken orally, 3 tablets each time, 3 times daily.

2) **Deficiency of both Qi and Yin**

Main Symptoms and Signs: Lassitude, languor, shortness of soft breath, flushed zygomatic region, dry mouth, restlessness, fever, night sweating, feverish sensation in the palms and soles, enlarged tender reddish tongue with exfoliative fur, and weak rapid pulse.

Therapeutic Principles: Tonifying both qi and yin.

Recipe:

Radix Panacis Quinquefolii	3 g
Radix Ophiopogonis	15 g
Fructus Schisandrae	
Radix Rehmanniae	12 g
Rhizoma Dioscoreae	12 g
Fructus Corni	12 g
Fructus Lycii	12 g
Cortex Eucommiae	9 g
Radix Angelicae Sinensis	9 g
Radix Glycyrrhizae Preparata	4.5 g

Decoct the above ingredients in a right amount of water for oral administration.

Modification: In case of flushed zygomatic region, and feverish sensation in the chest, palms and soles, the drugs added are *Radix Scrophulariae* 12 g, *Cortex Moutan* 12 g, *Cortex Lycii* 15 g, *Radix Cynanchi Atrati* 15 g.

Chinese Patent Medicine: *Baxian changshou wan* (*Eight – immortal longevity bolus*)

Indications: Yin – deficiency of the lung and kidney.

Administration: Taken orally, 9 g each time, twice daily.

3) **Yang – deficiency of the Spleen and Kidney**

Main Symptoms and Signs: Prolonged asthma, dyspnea, chills, cold limbs, poor appetite, loose stools, edema of the face and lower limbs, pale and enlarged tongue with white slippery coating, and deep thready pulse.

Therapeutic Principles: Warming and tonifying the spleen and kidney.

Recipe:

Radix Ginseng	3 g
Semen Juglandis	30 g
Radix Rehmanniae Praeparata	15 g
Rhizoma Dioscoreae	12 g
Fructus Lycii	12 g
Cortex Eucommiae	9 g
Fructus Corni	12 g
Fructus Schisandrae	6 g

Decoct the above ingredients in a right amount of water for oral administration.

Modification: In case of shortness of breath and dyspnea, the drugs added are *Radix Astragali* 30 g, *Lignum Aquilariae Resinatum* (taken after being infused in water) 1.5 g.

In case of edema, *Semen Plantaginis* (decocted after being wrapped in a piece of gauze) 30 g, *Talcum* 30 g and *Exocarpium Benincasae* 30 g are added.

Chinese Patent Medicine

1. *Ciwujia pian* (*Acanthopanax root tablet*)

Taken orally, 3 tablets each time, 3 times daily.

2. *Gejie dingchuan wan* (*Gecko pill for arresting asthma*)

Taken orally, 1.5 g each time, twice to 3 times daily.

PREVENTION

Prevent and cure with the above - stated methods the following primary diseases: cold, bronchitis, bronchial asthma, bronchiectasis and pulmonary tuberculosis.

Doing *Qigong*, abdominal - breathing and breathing - exercise plays a very important part in preventing the onset and development of this disease.

Chapter Fourteen
Pulmonary Abscess

Pulmonary abscess is a suppurative infection of the lung, is included in the category of syndrome of *lung carbuncle*, *feiyong* in traditional Chinese medicine. It is one kind of abscess developed due to pyogenic infection, necrosis and liquefaction in the lung, all of which are caused by various kinds of pathogenic bacteria such as *staphylococcus*, *streptococcus*, *diplococcus pneumoniae*, *fusiform bacillus*, *spirochete*, etc.. Clinically, it is characterized by high fever, cough and expectoration of profuse stink pyoid sputum.

ETIOLOGY AND PATHOGENESIS

This disease is resulted in due to deficiency of vital – qi, retention of phlegm – heat in the interior, affection of wind – cold which lasts long and produces heat, or attack by wind – heat pathogen. At the early stage, the pathogens have just started to attack the lung. Following that, heat – accumulation and blood stasis result. The combination of phlegm and blood stasis leads to the formation of carbuncle which develops into abscess when blood and flesh have been impaired into pus by the excessive noxious – heat. Timely and adequate treatment will cause the abscess to be festered, the noxious – heat to be released out of the body, the vital – qi to be restored, and the disease to be cured gradually. In the convalescence, yin – injury, qi – exhaustion and lingering noxious – heat may remain to different extent.

Pulmonary abscess is caused by a variety of pathogenic bacteria, most of which are anaerobe. The pathogens mostly invade the lung by aspiration. In a small percentage of patients the abscess arises from hematogenous infections.

MAIN POINTS OF DIAGNOSIS

1. **Medical history and onset of the disease**: Pulmonary abscess due to aspiration is frequently caused by vomit resulting from coma, drunken state and esophageal and pylonic obstruction, or by oral inflammation and pharyngolaryngeal operation. The pathogenic bacteria, carried into the lung through respiratory movements, multiply there. Hematogenous pulmonary abscess is often secondary to pyemia due to the pyogenic infections of the skin and deep tissues, osteomyelitis, etc..

2. **Clinical manifestations**: The onset is abrupt with initial symptoms of chills, fever,

chest pain, cough, hemoptysis and the production of a large amount of purulent sputum. The sputum is viscid and fetid. Standing for a while, three level may be seen. Sometimes the onset is insidious.

3. Physical examination: At the initial stage physical examination may show no obvious changes on the lung. When there is consolidation resulting from inflammation, there may be dullness on percussion. If there is a cavity formation, an amphoric sound may be elicited on percussion. Clubbing of the finger is noted on occasion. Weight loss and anemia are common.

4. In blood examination leukocyte count is markedly increased up to $20-30 \times 10^9$/L, increased neutrophil with a shift to left. In hematogenous pulmonary abscess blood culture may be positive and pathogenic bacteria can be identified. Bloody sputum culture and antimicrobial sensitive test should be done, which are helpful for selecting effective antibiotics. Chest X - ray examination is useful for discovering early lesions. Aspiration pulmonary abscess is mostly located in the posterior segment of the irght upper lobe and apical segment of the right lower lobe. At the initial stage there is a large area of consolidation. When abscess or abscess cavity is formed, fluid level within it can be seen. In hematogenous pulmonary abscess, many small dense shadows or globular shadows or thinwall cavities in both left and right middle and lower lobes may be present. computerized tomography is helpful in making correct diagnosis and in identifying the degree of involvement of the bronchi.

5. Sputum culture can reveal the etiology of the disease.

DIFFERENTIATION AND TREATMENT OF COMMON SYNDROMES

1. The Primary Stage

Main Symptoms and Signs: Chills, fever, cough, chest pain, small amount of mucous sputum, disturbance of breath, thin and yellowish coating of the tongue, floating and rapid pulse.

Therapeutic Principles: Clearing away and dispelling lung - heat and removing toxic substances from the lung.

Recipe 1:

Flos Lonicerae	30 g
Fructus Forsythiae	15 g
Folium Isatidis	15 g
Radix Scutellariae	12 g

Herba Taraxaci	30 g
Herba Menthae	10 g
Herba Houttuyniae	30 g
Bulbus Fritillariae Cirrhosae	10 g
Radix Platycodi	10 g

Decoct the above ingredients in a right amount of water for oral administration.

Attention should be paid to the cases complicated with chest pain, for which 20 grams of *Fructus Trichosanthis* and 12 grams of *Radix Curcumae* may be added.

Recipe 2:

Rhizoma Dryoperis Crassirhizomae	30 g
Folium Isatidis	15 g
Radix Arnebiae seu Lithospermi	15 g
Fructus Trichosanthis	12 g
Rhizoma Bistortae	15 g
Radix Platycodi	9 g
Radix Stemonae	9 g
Bulbus Fritillariae Thunbergii	9 g
Radix Trichosanthis	9 g
Exocarpium Citri Rubrum	9 g
Poria	9 g

Decoct the above ingredients in a right amount of water for oral administration.

Modification: In case of headache and general pain, the drugs added are *Folium Mori* 9 g, *Radix Puerariae* 15 g.

In case of severe chest pain, the drugs added are *Radix Salviae Miltiorrhizae* 12 g and *Radix Curcumae* 12 g and *Myrrha* 6 g.

In case of fullness in the chest and dyspnea, the drugs added are *Herba Ephedrae Praeparata* 9 g, *Semen Armeniacae Amarum* 9 g.

2. **The Abscess-forming Stage**

Main Symptoms and Signs: Fever, cough with dyspnea, chest fullness, chest pain, productive cough, polypnea, dry mouth without thirst, reddened tongue with yellow greasy fur, and smooth rapid pulse.

Therapeutic Principles: Removing pathogenic heat and toxic materials.

Recipe:

Rhizoma Phragmitis	30 g
Semen Coicis	30 g
Semen Benincasae	24 g

Semen Persicae 10 g
Flos Lonicerae 30 g
Fructus Forsythiae 15 g
Radix Scutellariae 12 g
Herba Houttuyniae 30 g
Fructus Trichosanthis 20 g
Radix Platycodi 10 g
Radix Glycyrrhizae 6 g

Decoct the above ingredients in a right amount of water for oral administration.

Apart from the above ingredients, 30 grams of *Gypsum Fibrosum* and 10 grams of *Rhizoma Anemarrhenae* are to be used for the patients with high fever and thirst; 30 grams of *Herba Taraxaci* , 15 grams of *Herba Violae* and 10 grams of *Fructus Gardeniae* for the cases with persisting high fever; 20 grams of *Radix Rehmanniae* and 12 grams of *Rhizoma Bletillae* for treating profuse hemoptysis; 12 grams of *Cortex Mori Radicis* and 10 grams of *Semen Lepidii seu Descurainiae* for overcoming profuse sputum and dyspnea with chest distention.

The Abscess – bursting Stage

Main Symptoms and Signs: Coughing out a large quantity of fetid and purulent sputum, sometimes mixed with blood, chest pain, stuffiness and distension in the chest, slow lysis fever, red tongue with yellow and greasy fur, deep and forceful or slippery and rapid pulse.

Therapeutic Principles: Draining pus and removing the poisonous substances.

Recipe:

Radix Platycodi 15 g
Semen coicis 20 g
Herba Houttuyniae 30 g
Herba Patriniae 30 g
Caulis Sargentodoxae 30 g
Semen Benincasae 30 g
Bulbus Fritillariae Thunbergii 15 g
Flos Lonicerae 30 g
Radix Glycyrrhizae 6 g

Decoct the above ingredients in a right amount of water for oral administration.

If the case at the restoration stage is accompanied with impaired qi and yin manifested by low fever, weakness, cough with little sputum, and expectorating persistently purulent blood, spontaneous perspiration and nightt sweat, red tongue with little fur, fine and rapid pulse, it is suitable to aim the treatment at nourishing qi and yin and clearing away the remaining poisonous substances. The chosen recipe is :

Modified prescriptions Decoction of Glehnia and Ophiopogon and Pulse – activating Powder

Radix Glehniae	15 g
Radix Ophiopogonis	15 g
Radix Pseudostellariae	12 g
Radix Astragali seu Hedysari	12 g
Semen Benincasae	20 g
Radix Platycodi	12 g
Rhizoma Bletillae	12 g
Radix Rehmanniae	15 g
Flos Lonicerae	15 g
Radix Glycyrrhizae Praeparata	6 g

4. **Recovery Stage**

Main Symptoms and Signs: The symptoms such as fever, cough and expectoration of purulent and bloody sputum become milder gradually, or are manifested by dull pain in the chest and hypochondium, shortness of breath, spontaneous perspiration, night sweat, low fever, tidal fever, pale complexion, emaciation, red or ligh – red tongue, thin, rapid and weak pulse.

Therapeutic Principles: Nourishing yin to tonify the lung and dispelling lingering toxins.

Recipe:

Radix Astragali	30 g
Radix Pseudostellariae	15 g
Semen Benincasae	15 g
Semen Coicis	15 g
Cortex Albiziae	15 g
Radix Glehniae	9 g
Rhizoma Bletillae	9 g
Radix Platycodi	9 g

Decoct the above ingredients in a right amount of water for oral administration.

Modification: In case of tidal fever after noon, the drugs added are *Cortex Lycii* 15 g, *Radix Cynanchi Atrati* 9 g, *Herba Artemisiae Annuae* 9 g.

In case of prolonged expectoration of foul thick turbid sputum, the drugs omitted are *Radix Glehniae*, *Rhizoma Bletillae*, the drugs added are *Rhizoma Fagopyri Cymosi*

30 g, *Herba Houttuyniae* 30 g, *Caulis Sargentodoxae* 30 g.

Chinese Patent Medicine: *Fufang yuxingcao pian* (*Composite pill of Houttuynia*)

Taken orally, 4 – 6 tablets each time, 3 times daily.

PREVENTION AND NURSING

Nursing

1) Encourage the patients to walk about but not over exert themselves.

2) Give the patients high calorie and high protein diet. The amount of food should be gradually increased but not be excessive so as to avoid damaging the stomach and spleen.

3) Since the period of disease is long and patient's mental burden is heavy, psycholigical nursing should be stressed to ease the patients' mind so as to benefit the recovery.

Prevention

Prevent actively acute or chronic inflammation in the mouth cavity or the upper respiratory tract, cavernous pulmonary tuberculosis, bronchiectasis complicated by infection, and aspiration pulmonary abscess; treat actively skin abrasion and infection, furuncle and carbuncle so as to prevent hematogenous lung abscess; nurse carefully the patients with coma and general anesthesia so as to prevent infection of the lung.

Chapter Fifteen
Pulmonary Tuberculosis

Pulmonary tuberculosis is an infectious disease due to infection of *tuberculosis bacillus* through the respiratory tract. It is classified into two types: primary and secondary and mainly manifested by cough, expectoration, hemoptysis, chest pain, tidal fever, night sweat and emaciation. It belongs to the category of *consumptive disease of the lung* in traditional Chinese medicine.

ETIOLOGY AND PATHOGENESIS

Tuberculosis bacillus attacks the lung and causes this disease when vital – qi is deficient. At the early stage, yin – fluid is usually exhausted and only the lung is involved. Following that, there occurs hyperactivity of fire due to yin – deficiency and both the lung and kidney are involved together with the heart and liver. Or both the spleen and lung are involved and both qi and yin are deficient. At the advanced stage, deficiency of yin affects yang, resulting in deficiency of both yin and yang. In the whole course, yin – deficiency is of the most importance.

DIFFERENTIATION AND TREATMENT OF COMMON SYNDROMES

1. Deficiency of the Lung – yin

Main Symptoms and Signs: Dry and brief cough, bright – red sputum streaked and spotted with blood, feverish sensation in the palms and soles after noon, dry and burning sensation in the skin, or mild night sweat, dry mouth and throat, vague dull pain in the chest, thin tongue coating, red tongue margin and tip, and thready or thready and rapid pulse.

Therapeutic Principles: Nourishing yin and moisturizing the lung.

Recipe:

Radix Asparagi	12 g
Radix Ophiopogonis	12 g
Radix Rehmanniae	15 g
Radix Rehmanniae Praeparata	15 g
Rhizoma Dioscoreae	24 g

Radix Stemonae 12 g
Radix Glehniae 12 g
Poria 12 g
Bulbus Fritillariae Cirrhosae 10 g
Liver of otter 12 g
Folium Mori 9 g
Flos Chrysanthemi 10 g
Colla Corii Asini 9 g
Radix Notoginseng 3 g

Decoct the above ingredients in a right amount of water for oral administration.

Modification: In case of sputum streaked with blood, the drugs added are *Rhizoma Bletillae* 12 g, *Herba Agrimoniae* 20 g, *Nodus Nelumbinis Rhizomatis* 12 g.

In case of low fever, the drugs added are *Radix Stellariae* 12 g, *cortex Lycii* 12 g, *Folium Mahoniae* 12 g and *Herba Artemisiae Annuae* 15 g.

2. Hyperactivity of Fire due to Yin – deficiency

Main Symptoms and Signs: Cough, dyspnea, scanty sticky or thick yellow sputum, frequent hemoptysis with bright red blood, tidal fever after noon, bone – heat, severe feverish sensation in the chest, palms and soles, flushed cheeks, night sweat, thirst, restlessness, insomnia, impatience, irritability, pain in the chest and hypochondrium, impotence in male, irregular menstruation in female, gradual emaciation, deep red and dry tongue with thin yellow coating, and thready rapid pulse.

Therapeutic Principles: Nourishing yin and reduce fire.

Recipe:

Bulbus Lilii 30 g
Radix Ophiopogonis 12 g
Radix Scrophulariae 15 g
Radix Rehmanniae Praeparata 15 g
Radix Rehmanniae 15 g
Carapax Trionycis 24 g
Rhizoma Anemarrhenae 9 g
Radix Gentianae Macrophyllae 12 g
Herba Artemisiae Annuae 12 g
Radix Angelicae Sinensis 9 g
Radix Paeoniae Alba 12 g
Radix Stellariae 12 g
Radix Platycodi 9 g

Fructus Mume 6 g
Cortex Lycii 12 g
Radix Glycyrrhizae 6 g

Decoct the above ingredients in a right amount of water for oral administration.

Modification: For profuse yellow sputum, the drugs added are ***Cortex Mori*** 9 g, ***Fructus Aristolochiae*** 9 g, ***Herba Houttuyniae*** 30 g.

In case of persistent hemoptysis, the drugs added are ***Cortex Moutan*** 12 g, ***Fructus Gardeniae*** 9 g, ***Carbonized Radix et Rhizoma Rhei*** 9 g, ***Herba Callicarpae Pedunculatae*** 12 g.

In case of hemoptysis with dark purple blood, the drugs added are ***Radix Notoginseng*** 3 g, ***Crinis Carbonisatus*** 10 g, ***Ophicalcitum*** 20 g and ***Radix Curcumae*** 10 g.

For night sweat, the drugs added are ***Fructus Mume*** 12 g, ***forged Os Draconis Fossilia*** 30 g, ***forged Choncha Ostreae*** 30 g and ***Fructus Tritici Levis*** 12 g.

For hoarse voice or aphonia, the drugs added are ***Fructus Chebulae*** 10 g, ***Membrana Follicularis Ovi*** 10 g, ***Semen Juglandis*** 10 g and ***Mel*** 10 g.

3. Exhaustion and Impairment of Qi and Yin

Main Symptoms and Signs: Cough, weakness, shortness of breath, languor, sputum sometimes with light red blood, mild tidal fever after noon, pale complexion, flushed cheeks, reddened tender tongue with thin white coating and tooth-prints on the margin, and thready weak and rapid pulse.

Therapeutic Principles: Invigorating qi and nourishing yin.

Recipe:

Radix Codonopsis 18 g
Radix Astragali 24 g
Rhizoma Atractylodis Macrocephalae 10 g
Poria 12 g
Radix Asparagi 12 g
Radix Ophiopogonis 12 g
Radix Rehmanniae 15 g
Radix Rehmanniae Praeparata 15 g
Radix Angelicae Sinensis 12 g
Radix Paeoniae Rubra 15 g
Radix Paeoniae Alba 15 g
Cortex Phellodendri 6 g
Rhizoma Anemarrhenae 6 g
Cortex Magnoliae Officinalis 6 g

Fructus Schisandrae	6 g
Radix Bupleuri	6 g
Pericarpium Citri Reticulatae	9 g
Plumula Nelumbinis	3 g
Cortex Lycii	12 g
Rhizoma Zingiberis Recens	6 g
Radix Glycyrrhizae	6 g
Fructus Jujubae	5 dates

Decoct the above ingredients in a right amount of water for oral administration.

Modification: For dilute sputum, the drugs added are *Radix Asteris* 12 g, *Flos Farfarae* 12 g, *Fructus Perillae* 12 g.

For hemoptysis, the drugs added are *Colla Corii Asini* 12 g, *Herba Agrimoniae* 20 g, *Radix Notoginseng* (in the form of powder) 3 g.

For bone - heat and night sweat, the drugs added are *Carapax Trionycis* 10 g, *Concha Ostreae* 30 g and *Radix Stellariae* 12 g.

For abdominal distention, loose stools and poor appetite, the drugs added are *Semen Lablab Album* 12 g, *Semen Coicis* 30 g and *Semen Nelumbinis* 20 g.

4. Deficiency of both Yin and Yang

Main Symptoms and Signs: Cough, dyspnea, sputum soetimes with dark red blood, tidal fever, chills, spontaneous sweating, night sweat, hoarse voice, aphonia, edema of the face and limbs, palpitation, purple lips, cold limbs, diarrhea before dawn, aphthous stomatitis, extreme emaciation, spermatorrhea and impotence in male, scanty menstruation or amenia in female, reddened and dry tongue or pale enlarged tongue with tooth - prints on the margin, and indistinct thready rapid or feeble large pulse.

Therapeutic Principles: Nourishing yin and reinforcing yang.

Recipe:

Radix Codonopsis	18 g
Radix Astragali	24 g
Rhizoma Dioscoreae	24 g
Fructus Lycii	15 g
Carapax et Plastrum Testudnis	30 g
Cornu Cervi	6 g
Radix Angelicae Sinensis	12 g
Radix Paeoniae Alba	12 g
Radix Rehmanniae Praeparata	15 g
Placenta Hominis	15 g

Rhizoma Atractylodis Macrocephalae 9 g

Poria 12 g

Decoct the above ingredients in a right amount of water for oral administration.

Modification: In case of dyspnea, the drugs added are *Cordyceps* 10 g, *Fructus Chebulae* 10 g and *Stalactitum* 20 g.

For palpitation, the drugs added are *Fluoritum* 20 g, *Radix Salviae Miltiorrhizae* 30 g.

For diarrhea before dawn, the drugs added are *roasted Semen Myristicae* 12 g and *Fructus Psoraleae* 12 g.

Simple Prescription:

Zaocys proper amount

Administration: The drug is boiled until its crust chars with its original properties retained, taken with boiled water after meal, 9 g each time, 3 times daily.

Indications: Pulmonary tuberculosis with the symptoms of low fever, night sweat and severe debility, or tuberculosis of lymph nodes.

Precautions: Smaller dosage is used for young children.

Proven Prescription:

Cacumen Platycladi 90 g

Rhizoma Zingiberis 90 g

Folium Artemisiae Argyi 60 g

brown sugar proper amount

The first three ingredients are decocted in 1500 ml of water until 500 ml of the decoction can be got. The 500 ml of decoction is mixed with *brown sugar* into a mixture. 60 ml of the mixture is taken each time, 4 – 6 times a day.

Indications: Hemoptysis due to pulmonary tuberculosis.

Chinese Patent Medicine: *Mai wei dihuang wan* (*Eight – immortals Longevity bolus*).

Administration: Taken with warm boiled water, one bolus each time, twice daily.

PREVENTION

1. Conduct vaccination of bacille *Calmette Guerin* to strengthen the resistance against mycobacterium buberculosis and lower the incidence of the disease.

2. Make periodic health examinations so as to diagnose and treat the disease at its early stage.

3. Follow strictly the rules for the administration and isolation of tuberculosis and the principles for disinfection.

Chapter Sixteen
Cancer of Lung

Cancer of lung (pulmonary carcinoma, primary bronchopulmonary carcinoma, PBC) is one of the most common malignant tumors. In this century, the rate of incidence in many countries has soared. Its morbidity and mortality rates are comparatively high. For those patients who are post – middle aged, heavy smokers or who suffer from chronic bronchitis, the morbidity rate is quite high. This indicates serious environmental polution is a n important etiological factor. The incidence among smokers is 10 to 40 times higher than for non – smokers. Lack of vitamin A and C in food, weakness of the body's anticancer factor and psychic trauma lowers the immune function, increasing sensitivity to canceration.

Pulmonary carcinoma is classified as central and peripheral type, according to location of the lesion. It can also be divided according to morphological characteristics, intratubal, tube wall, globula, huge mass and diffused type. Histological classification shows: squamous carcinoma 40% to 43%; adenocarcinoma 37% to 42%; undifferentiated carcinoma 13% to 17%, including small and large cell carcinoma, and bronchiolo – alveolar carcinoma 2% to 5%.

In traditional Chinese medicine, pulmonary carcinoma belongs to the categories of *chest pain*, *xi ben*, *asthma*, *lung accumulation*, *mass and lumps*, *cough*, *hemoptysis* and *thoracalgia*. Its causes and mechanisms are summarized as the invasion of pathogenic factors into lungs, the dwelling of phlegm – dampness in the interior, or the deficiency of both qi and yin in lung.

ETIOLOGY AND PATHOGENESIS

The disease is all due to deficiency. Deficiency here mainly means both qi and yin deficiency of the lung. It is deficiency that invites attack of pathogens or results in accumulation of phlegm – dampness in the interior. Long stagnation of phlegm – dampness and noxious pathogens in the lung leads to the formation of masses. This disease belongs to the type ***deficiency in origin and excess in superficiality***. Deficiency is the cause, while excess the manifestations. Deficiency is general, while excess localized.

CLINICAL MANIFESTATIONS

1. Symptoms of Pulmonary Carcinoma

Symptoms manifested are similar to common pulmonary ailments and difficult to differentiate. The early or late appearance of symptoms, and their severity reflect the location of the neoplasm and its degree of development. The symptoms of central type appear early and the peripheral type late. Common symptoms are as follows:

1) **Cough**: The most common feature by far is initially the cough, particularly in the central type. It is the outstanding feature. The characteristic pulmonary cancer cough is an irritating non-productive cough, with only smal amounts of white, foaming mucinous sputum. If the neoplasm is located at the general bronchus or in the vicinity of prominence, the cough will be more vigorous, and antitussives are ineffective. There is no cough or only a mild cough displayed when the neoplasm locates in the mucous membrane of bronchiole. The cough of PBC is usually covered by a cough from chronic bronchitis or heavy smoking. If the nature or pattern of ordinary coughing suddenly changes, the possibility of PBC should be considered.

2) **Hemoptysis or Spitting Bloody Sputum**: Hemoptysis is a common feature of PC. It occurs mainly when the neoplasm located in the bronchial mucosa ruptures and bleeds, and is often observed in the central type PC. Its characteristic is intermittent small amounts of bloody sputum, fresh blood predominating over sputum. Coptious hemoptysis seldom occurs. The persistence of hemoptysis is different, as it usually lasts a few days, then stops spontaneously without treatment. It can also last for months, and is difficult to stop even with hemostatics. It usually occurs in central type PC with central necrosis and lysis accompanied by bleeding.

3) **Fever**: The complaint of many patients is recurrent fever, self-diagnosed as a common cold or bronchitis and PC is discovered when they seek a doctor's advice. Half of such patients are then diagnosed as having a bronchial infection or segmental pneumonia. Although the symptoms improve after treatment, absorption of the lesion is incomplete, or reappears many times. When a detailed investigation is made, a diagnosis of PC is finally established. Causes of the fever are: obstruction of bronchus, secretion from the infection stgnates and becomes re-infected; another cause is pyrogen or metabolite released from the neoplasm which stimulates the thermoregulatory center and causes fever. The first type can be treated effectively with anti-phlogistic therapy, while it is necessary to use indomethason, butazolidin and corticoid to bring down the fever of the second type.

4) **Chest Pain**: Chest pain is a characteristic feature of PC. Dull chest pain in a fixed location usually reflects the focus site of the carcinoma below it. Persistent, severe, sharp

pain indicates the pleura, chest wall and ribs are invaded, it frequently occurs in small cell carcinoma of the lungs. Wandering or fixed pain of systemic muscles and skeleton without positive findings after physical examination, are due to stimulation from the cancers toxin in advanced stage.

5) Dyspnea: Tumor grows at the inlet of bronchus and obstructs its lumen which causes disturbance of ventilation and atelectasis. It manifests itself as dyspnea or shortness of breath. This symptom occurs when there is metastasis to pleura complicated pleural effusion.

2. Symptoms of Tumor Compression and Metastasis

When the neoplasm compresses or involves the recurrent nerve, paralysis of vocal cords occurs. As the neoplasm compresses and invades the upper vena caba, vertigo, blurred vision, distress in the chest, edema of the head, neck, chest and back occurs, and dilation of cutaneous capillaries appears. Dysphagia occurs if it spreads to the mediastinum and compresses the esophagus; In Horner's syndrome the affected side manifests as enophthalmus, ptosis of eyelid, miosis, narrowing of palpebral fissure, and skin temperature of upper half of chest and face increase.

Anhydrosis appears when the malignant tumor invades C_7 and the lateral of T_1. Intracranial hypertensive symptoms such as headache, vertigo, and vomiting appear after the brain is involved. Metastases to pleura and pericardium cause effusion which is manifested by chest distree, and dyspnea, heart sounds become low and distant, diminution of respiration on affected side, and dullness on percussion. In advanced stage of skeletal metastasis, severe ostealgia appears. Paraplegia occurs as the neoplasm spreads to vertebra and compresses the spinal cord. When it extends to the liver symptoms of liver carcinoma appear. In advanced stage of pulmonary carcinoma, the outcome is complicated mainly by infection, disturbance in respiration, and overburdening the heart, causing heart failure.

MAIN POINTS OF DIAGNOSIS

Interrogate and obtain the history in detail, adding the previously mentioned details of symptoms as well as laboratory findings helpful to establish an early diagnosis.

1. X-ray Examination

It is very important to use X-ray for the diagnosis of pulmonary carcinoma, as it has a definite value. Roentgenological investigation should be carried out according to the conditions and need. X-ray examination reflects only local pathological changes. It is necessary to supplement with other investigations to assure a comprehensive analysis and correct diagnosis.

2. **To Find Tumor Cells in Cytological Study from Sputum**

The advantage of this method is easy access to sputum samples, and the fact it can be repeated without causing the patient to suffer. When the sample is collected properly, and examination technique is skillful, positivity can exceed 75%. Before collecting the sample, have the patient gargle, clean mouth, and expectorate out all saliva and sputum accumulated in the throat, then cough vigorously, and expectorate from the bottom of the lungs three or four times. Put sputum in a clear bottle with wide opening and submit immediately for examination. Using the bloody-streaked, fine granules or white filiform portions of the sputum can help obtain a higher positivity.

3. **Fiberbronchoscopy**

Using fiberbronchoscopy, the status of the vocal cords can be observed, and if there is ulceration, rigidness, obstruction, compression in the trachea and large bronchus; or whether the prominance has become wide, is fixed or displaced. Secretion for a smear, can be obtained to determine indications for surgery and help formulate a program for treatment and is a valuable means for diagnosis and differential diagnosis.

4. **CT Examination**

This is an important measure todetermine tumor's relationship to surrounding tissues, its location and size; to observe if there are metastases to mediastinal lymph nodes and the contralateral lung; and to decide the therapeutic procedure.

5. **Other Examinations**

When necessary, mediastinoscopy, and iotope scanning of lungs can be supplemented as diagnostic measures. Laboratory findings such as ESR, enzymatic examination, value of β-fetal protein may increase, but will have no specific significance for the diagnosis of pulmonary carcinoma.

DIFFERENTIATION AND TREATMENT OF COMMON SYNDROMES

Different syndromes are revealed which depend on varying situations of conflict between the body resistance and pathogenic factors, also if the patient's constitution is sthenia or asthenia. Method of typing has not yet been unified domestically, but different typings are actually similar, with only minor differences.

1. **Lung Heat and Yin Deficiency Type**

Most patients belong to the central type of pulmonary carcinoma, with recurrent involvement of laryngeal nerve or complicated by infection.

Main Symptoms and Signs: Dry irritating cough, without or with sparse sticky sputum, occasional bloody sputum, accompanied by low fever, night sweating, chest distress, dry throat, hoarseness, irritability, insomnia, dry mouth and thirst, red or red-purple tongue with thin yellow or white coating, faint and quick pulse.

Therapeutic Principles: Nourishing yin and moistening lung, clearing up the evil heat and inhibiting the cancer.

Recipe:

Radix Glehniae	15 g
Radix Ophiopogonis	15 g
Radix Asparagi	15 g
Cortex Lycii	12 g
Bulbus Lilii	12 g
Radix Scutellariae	10 g
Herba Dendrobii	12 g
Fructus Trichosanthis	24 g
Bulbus Fritillariae Cirrhosae	9 g
Carapax Trionycis	15 g
Herba Oldenlandiae Diffusae	24 g
Herba Scutellariae Barbarae	24 g
Herba Houtuyniae	24 g
Rhizoma Gynostemmatis Pentaphylli	15 g

Add or subtract drugs according to syndrome differentiation.

2. Stagnancy of Phlegm and Dampness in Lung

Most belong to tubal wall type or central type of bronchial carcinoma, with bronchial infection, or superior vena cava syndrome.

Main Symptoms and Signs: Productive cough, with white, thin sputum, flatulence and anorexia, weakness of limbs, normal or loose stool, edema of head, face and chest, subcutaneous vascular dilation in neck and upper thoracic region, white tongue with white greasy coating, slippery and quick pulse.

Therapeutic Principles: Supplement qi and strengthen the spleen, dispel the phlegm and dampness.

Recipe:

Radix Codonopsis	15 g
Rhizoma Atractylodis Macrocephalae	12 g
Poria	12 g
Radix Glycyrrhizae	3 g
Semen Plantaginis	12 g

Rhizoma Dioscoreae 15 g
Rhizoma Pinelliae 9 g
Pericarpium Citri Reticulatae 9 g
Radix Peucedani 9 g
Polyporus 18 g
Semen Armeniaca Amarum 9 g
Bulbus Fritillariae Cirrhosae 9 g
Rhizoma Alismatis 6 g
Semen Coicis 18 g
Radix Asteris 10 g
Semen Euryales 15 g

Add or subtract drugs according to syndrome differentiation.

3. Deficiency of Qi in both the Spleen and Lung

Main Symptoms and Signs: Sallow complexion, emaciation, scant food intake, fatigue, shortness of breath, forceless cough; accompanied by slight expectoration, stagnated blood in the tongue (often seen in adenocarcinoma).

Recipe:

Radix Astragali seu hedysari 10 g
Radix Codonopsis Pilosulae 10 g
Poria 10 g
Rhizoma Atractylodis Macrocephalae 10 g
Semen Coicis 10 g
Rhizoma Pinelliae 10 g
Pericarpium Metaplexis Japonici 10 g
Fructus Viticis Negundo 10 g
Radix et Cortex Eaomynus Grandiflori 10 g
Rhizoma Ligustici Chuanxiong 10 g
Radix Ranunculi Ternati 15 g
Pericarpium Citri Reticulatae 5 g

4. Deficiency of both Qi and Yin

Main Symptoms and Signs: Dry cough with no phlegm or little sputum mixed with blood streaks, low fever, burning sensation in the palms and soles, night sweating, shortness of breath, dry mouth, constipation, dark-reddish tongue with little or no fur, thin-rapid or thin-taut pulse; dizziness, tinnitus, emaciation, little appetite, fatigue, sublingual phlebectasis. *This type is often seen in adenocarcinoma and undifferentiated carcinoma.*

Recipe:

Radix Pseudostellariae	10 g
Radix Glehniae	10 g
Radix Asparagi	10 g
Radix Ophiopogonis	10 g
Bulbus Lilii	10 g
Rhizoma Polygonati Odorati	10 g
Rhizoma Dioscoreae	10 g
Rhizoma Polygonati	10 g
Cortex Moutan Radicis	10 g
Radix Paeoniae Rubra	10 g
Semen Persicae	10 g
Herba Ecliptae	10 g
Cortex Lycii Radicis	10 g
Folium Mahoniae	10 g
Radix Ginseng	6 g

Modification: If pressed superior vena cava syndrome is present in all the above types, *Semen Lepidii seu Descurainiae* 10 – 15 g, *Polyporus Umbellatus* 15 – 30 g, *Herba Ephedrae* 10 g added for hemoptysis. *Pollen Typhae* 10 – 15 g, *Herba Eragrostis Cilianensis* 30 – 60 g added and the drugs for promoting blood circulation stopped. In case of severe chest pain, *Rhizoma Corydalis* (ground into powder) 3 – 6 g and *Moschus* 0.2 g added (The two drugs dissolved in the decoction to be taken twice orally).

5. Blood Stasis with Evil Heat

Advanced stage of pulmonary carcinoma accompanied with infection, with invasion of pleura, rib or remote metastasis, sometimes exhibits hydrothorax and atelectasis.

Main Symptoms and Signs: Hard cough, sputum yellow or bloody, chest distress and pain, or accompanied with pain of entire body, definite or indefinite locations, fever at times, constipation, dry mouth, dark crimson tongue with petechiae, thick or thin yellow coating, tense, wiry, thready and uneven pulse.

Therapeutic Principles: Detoxicating and resolving the stasis, clearing up the evil heat and nourishing yin.

Recipe:

Flos Lonicerae	10 g
Rhizoma Paridis	15 g
Radix Paeoniae Rubra	12 g

Poria	15 g
Radix Ophiopogonis	15 g
Rhizoma Imperatae	15 g
Herba Agrimoniae	30 g
Herba Dendrobii	12 g
Rhizoma Anemarrhenae	12 g
Gypsum Fibrosum	30 g
Radix Pseudostellariae	15 g
Fructus Akebiae	12 g
Herba Solanii Lyrati	10 g
Herba Oldenlandiae Diffusae	20 g
Herba Houttuyniae	20 g
Rhizoma et Radix Rhei	9 g
Fructus Trichosanthis	18 g

Add or subtract according to syndrome differentiation.

6. **Deficiency of both Spleen and Kidney**

At advanced stage of the disease, general debility due to the prolonged course, pulmonary ventilatory function is decreased and syndromes of lung and heart appear.

Main Symptoms and Signs: Chest distress and shortness of breath, cough and dyspnea aggravated during exertion, unable to expectorate, pale complexion, lumbago and weakness, anorexia, occasional hectic fever and spontaneous sweating, thready pulse, pink or dull color tongue with thin yellow or white coating.

Therapeutic Principles: Nourishing the kidney and lungs, strengthening body resistance and inhibiting the cancer.

Recipe:

Radix Pseudostellariae	15 g
Poria	15 g
Fructus Lycii	12 g
Radix Astragali	15 g
Rhizoma Atractylodis Macrocephalae	12 g
Fructus Schisandrae	6 g
Fructus Corni	9 g
Radix Ginseng	6 g
Rhizoma Polygonati	12 g
Semen Armeniaca Amarum	9 g
Radix Glycyrrhizae	3 g

Pericarpium Citri Reticulatae 8 g
Bulbus Fritilariae Cirrhosae 9 g
Herba Oldenlandiae Diffusae 20 g
Cordyceps 6 g

Add or subtract drugs according to existing symptoms.

The types mentioned above are the summarization of common clinical symptoms and pathogenesis of pulmonary carcinoma. They could be subdivided into many types, the type of syndrome varying with the changing condition of the patient. A type seldom exists in isolation. Differential treatment should therefore not be limited to these mentioned types in clinical practice.

7. Block of Stagnant Blood in Lung

Main Symptoms and Signs: Dark complexion, dark – purplish tongue or with ecchymoses, sublingual venous engorgement, accompanied by miliary hyperplasia, fixed thoracalgia; accompanied by cough, expectoration, bloody sputum, feeling of stuffiness in the chest and difficulty in breathing, scant food intake, lack of strength, emaciation, deep and uneven pulse. *This type is usually seen in squamous – cell carcinoma, adenocarcinoma and undifferentiated carcinoma.*

Recipe:

Radix et Cortex Eaomynus grandiflori 10 g
Pericarpium Trichosanthis 10 g
Radix Curcumae 10 g
Rhizoma Atractylodis Macrocephalae 10 g
Semen Coicis 10 g
Radix Ranunculi Ternati 15 g
Carapax Trionycis 15 g
Lignum Sappan 15 g
Radix Ginseng 6 g
Fructus Ziziphi Jujubae 5 pieces

Decoct the above ingredients in a right amount of water for oral administration.

8. Combination of Phlegm Turbidity and Blood Stagnancy

Main Symptoms and Signs: Cough with moderate sticky sputum white or yellow – white in color, feeling of stuffiness in the chest and difficulty with breathing, yellow – greasy or thick and yellow – greasy coating, string – like or taut and smoothy pulse, accompanied by dark tongue with ecchymoses, stuffiness in chest and thoracalgia, scanty ingestion, alck of strength and emaciation. Most of the cases had history of chronic bronchitis. *This type is often seen in squamous – cell carcinoma.*

Recipe:

Radix Ranunculi Ternati 15 g

Rhizoma Dioscoreae Bulbiferae	10 g
Semen Lepidii seu Descurainiae	10 g
Bulbus Fritillariae	10 g
Pericarpium Metaplexis Japonici	10 g
Concha Meretricis seu Cyclinae	10 g
Semen Persicae	10 g
Eupolyphaga seu Steleophaga	10 g
Radix Astragali seu Hedysari	10 g
Radix Codonopsis Pilosulae	10 g
Rhizoma Atractylodis Macrocephalae	10 g
Semen Coicis	10 g

9. Stagnation of Qi and Blood

Main Symptoms and Signs: Difficulty in expectoration, sputum with blood, localized chest pain, dyspnea, constipation, dark purple lips and nails, tongue with purplish ecchymoses or scattered patechiae, thin or yellow tongue coating, and taut or uneven pulse.

Therapeutic Principles: Promoting the circulation of both qi and blood to remove blood stasis and soften masses.

Recipe:

Radix Angelicae Sinensis	12 g
Radix Rehmanniae	15 g
Semen Persicae	10 g
Flos Carthami	10 g
Radix Paeoniae Rubra	12 g
Fructus Aurantii	10 g
Radix Bupleuri	12 g
Radix Trichosanthis	15 g
Semen Trichosanthis	30 g
Squama Manitis Praeparata	12 g
Spica Prunellae	15 g
Sargassum	30 g

Decoct the above ingredients in a right amount of water for oral administration.

Modification: In case of sputum with profuse blood, the drugs added are *Herba Curcurliginis* 30 g, *Cacumen Platycladi* 15 g and *Herba Scutellariae Barbatae* 30 g.

In case of profuse sputum which is difficult to expectorate out, the drugs added are *Os costaziae* 15 g, *parched Smen Armeniacae Amarum* 9 g, *Semen Lepidii seu Descurainiae* 9 g and *Radix Asteris* 12 g

10. **Phlegm – dampness Obstruction**

Main Symptoms and Signs: More severe cough with profuse sticky or puric sputum, choking pain in the chest, anorexia, loose stools, fever, deep colored urine, yellow and greasy tongue coating, and slippery rapid pulse.

Therapeutic Principles: Clearing away heat, resolving phlegm, inducing diuresis and removing toxic material.

Recipe:

Aresaema cum Bile	10 g
Rhizoma Pinelliae Praeparata	10 g
Poria	15 g
Pericarpium Citri Reticulatae	10 g
Cortex Mori	15 g
Herba Houttuyniae	30 g
Radix Peucedani	10 g
Fructus Aristolochiae	10 g
Semen Coicis	30 g
Cortex Magnoliae Officinalis	10 g
Herba Hedyotis Diffusae	30 g
Herba Scutellariae Barbatae	30 g
Rhizoma Smilacis Glabrae	30 g

Decoct the above ingredients in a right amount of water for oral administration.

Modification: In case of hydrothorax, dyspnea and choking sensation, the drugs added are *Semen Lepidii seu Descurainiae* 12 g, *Fructus Jujubae* 7 dates.

In case of pain in the chet and back, the drugs added are *Rhizoma Corydalis* 9 g, *Radix Stephaniae Tetrandrae* 9 g, *Olibanum* 12 g, *Myrrha* 12 g and *Scorpio* 9 g.

11. **Noxious – heat due to Deficiency of Yin**

Main Symptoms and Signs: Cough without or with little sputum or with bloody sputum, hemoptysis in severe cases, chest pain, restlessness, insomnia, low fever, night sweat, or high fever lasting longer, thirst, constipation, reddened tongue with thin yellow coating, and thready rapid or rapid large pulse.

Therapeutic Principles: Nourishing yin, clearing away heat, removing toxic material and resolving masses.

Recipe:

Radix Glehniae	30 g
Radix Ophiopogonis	15 g
Rhizoma Poligonati Odorati	15 g

Herba Dendrobii 30 g
Semen Armeniacae Amarum 10 g
Bulbus Fritillariae Cirrhosae 10 g
Radix Trichosanthis 15 g
Radix Asteris Praeparata 10 g
Concha Meretricis seu Cyclinae 30 g
Fructus Trichosanthis 30 g
Herba Taraxaci 30 g
Herba Scutellariae Barbatae 30 g
Rhizoma Bistortae 30 g

Decoct the above ingredients in a right amount of water for oral administration.

Modification: In case of persistent hemoptysis, the drugs added are *Herba Agrimoniae* 30 g, *Rhizoma Imperatae* 30 g, *Radix Rubae* 15 g and *Radix Notoginseng* 10 – 15 g.

In case of constipation, the drugs added are *Radix et Rhizoma Rhei* 6 g, *Radix Rehmanniae* 15 g, *Radix Scrophulariae* 15 g, *Semen Pruni* 15 g and *Fructus Cannabis* 12 g.

12. Deficiency of both Qi and Yin

Main Symptoms and Signs: Weak cough with little thin sticky sputum, shortness of breath, dyspnea, lassitude, acratia, pale complexion, emaciation, aversion to wind, spontaneous sweating or night sweat, dry mouth with little desire for drink, reddened or pale tongue, and thready weak pulse.

Therapeutic Principles: Invigorating qi, nourishing yin, clearing away heat and resolving phlegm.

Recipe:

Radix Codonopsis 30 g
Radix Ophiopogonis 15 g
Radix Glehniae 15 g
Rhizoma Dioscoreae 15 g
Fructus Schisandrae 6 g
Bulbus Fritillariae Cirrhosae 10 g
Fructus Trichosanthis 15 g
Spica Prunellae 15 g
Pseudobulbus Cremastrae seu Pleiones 15 g

Decoct the above ingredients in a right amount of water for oral administration.

Modification: In case of the disorder involving both the lung and kidney and with yang – deficiency more evident, the drugs added are *Rhizoma Curculiginis* 10 g, *Herba Epemedii* 15 g, *Herba Cistanches* 10 g, *Radix Morindae Officinalis* 15 g and *Fructus Psoraleae* 30 g.

In case of more severe deficiency of yin, the drugs added are *Radix Asparagi* 15 g, *Radix Rehmanniae* 15 g, *Radix Scrophulariae* 15 g, *Rhizoma Polygonati* 10 g and *Carapax et Plastrum Testudinis* 30 g.

If there is mass in the neck, the drugs added are *Radix Ranunculus Ternati* 15 g, *Pseudobulbus Cremastrae seu Pleiones* 15 g, *Spica Prunellae* 30 g, *Rhizoma Bolbostemmae* 12 g and *Squama Manitis* 15 g.

Chinese Patent Medicine: *Xi huang wan* (*Bolus of Rhinoceros horn and Cow – bezoar*)

Administration: Taken with warm boiled water, one bolus each time, twice daily.

13. Approved Prescription

Herba Houttuyniae	24 g
Poria	15 g
Polyporus	15 g
Radix Glehniae	15 g
Radix Ophiopogonis	9 g
Bulbus Fritillariae Cirrhosae	9 g
Radix Asteris	9 g
Flos Farfarae	9 g
Rhizoma Gynostemmatis Pentaphylli	15 g
Herba Agrimoniae	30 g
Radix Ginseng	6 g
Radix Pseudostellariae	15 g
Flos Lonicerae	10 g
Fructus Trichosanthis	20 g
Radix Glycyrrhizae	3 g
Herba Oldenlandiae Diffusae	24 g
Herba Solanii Lyrti	30 g

Decoct the above ingredients in a right amount of water for oral administration.

14. **Drugs Added or Subtracted According to Differentiation**1) Fever with chest pain or pantalgia, leucocytosis: *Radix Scutellariae* and *Herba Artemisiae Annuae* are selected to add in the prescription.

2) Constipation, dry mouth, crimson tongue and irritability: *Radix et Rhizoma Rhei* 9 to 12 g, *Folium Sennae* 9 g, *Radix Anemarrhenae* 12 g, *Herba Dendrobii* 15 g are added, with *Succus Bambusae* one ampule, 2 times daily.

3) Expectorate yellow sputum with difficulty, sometimes with hemoptysis: Add *Caulis Bambusae in Taeniam* 10 g, *Radix Platycodi* 10 g, *Succus Bambusae* 1-2 ampules and *Rhizoma Imperatae* 15 g in the prescription.

4) Superior vena cava syndrome: Add *Radix Salviae Miltiorrhizae* 15 g, *Herba Prunellae* 15 g, *Semen Plantaginis* 12 g and *Radix Pseudostellariae* 15 g.

5) Hydrothorax: Add *Semen Plantaginis* 15 g, *Semen Lepidii* 12 g, *Cortex Mori* 10 g and *Folium Eriobotryae* 12 g.

TREATMENT INTEGRATING TCM AND MODERN MEDICINE

Surgery, radiotherapy, chemotherapy and traditional Chinese Medicine are still the major means for treating pulmonary carcinoma. Methods should be selected according to the stage, and the progress of the disease. Traditional Chinese medicine for strengthening of the body resistance and western medicine for inhibiting the neoplasm should be full utilized. Comprehensive application of both medicines should be used to escalate the efficacy.

1. Principle of Treatment

1) Occult Carcinoma: Cancer cells are found in bronchial secretion in this types, but X-ray film and fiberbronchoscopy do not reveal the carcinoma focus. TCM is used to strengthen body resistance, clear up the evil heat, detoxicate, and balance the yin and yang.

2) Early and Middle Stage of Squamous Carcinoma and Adenocarcinoma: No matter which stage, early or late, or whether radiotherapy or chemotherapy are being used or not, TCM should be an adjuvant treatment under all these circumstances.

3) Stage Ⅲ: The patient should be treated non-surgical initially with combined therapy of TCM and modern medicine.

4) Stage Ⅳ: Mainly systemic, comprehensive therapy of TCM and modern medicine should be given.

2. Surgery

Treatment according to the patient's condition, requires one or more of the five operations which follow: pulmonary lobectomy, total pneumonectomy, pulmonary lobectomy and sleeve resection of bronchus, or/and bronchotomoplasty and palliative resection may be selected.

1) Pre-operative Adjustment by TCM and Modern Medicine: Weakened body resistance complicated by infection (stagnancy of the evil-heat) is the chief factor that cause post-operative complications and death. Measures for strengthening body resistance, eliminating the evil-heat and adjusting the internal imbalance of yin and yang are of great

importance. The TCM prescription commonly used is:

Radix Ophiopogonis	10 g
Radix Glehniae	10 g
Flos Lonicerae	10 g
Poria	12 g
Radix Psuedostellariae	15 g
Herba Houttuyniae	20 g
Folium Eriobotryae	10 g
Radix Platycodi	10 g
Radix Asteris	9 g
Bulbus Fritillariae Cirrhosae	8 g
Caulis Bambusae in Taeniam	10 g
Polyporus	15 g
Fructus Schisandrae	6 g
Herba Oldenlandiae Diffusae	24 g
Radix Astragali	15 g

Add or subtract drugs according to syndrome differentiation.

This prescriptin takes into account the characteristics of bronchial carcinoma: yin-deficiency, bronchial infection and declining immune function. It strengthens body resistance, nourishes yin, clears up the evil heat, disolves the phlegm and relieves coughing to create favorable conditions for surgery.

2) Post-operative Adjustment Using TCM and Modern Medicine: Injury and stress caused by surgery not only weakens the resistance of the organism against disease, but also cause the appearance of yin-deficiency or eil heat syndrome. Adjuvant therapy based on syndrome differentiation for strengthening body resistance and nourishing yin, is necessary and should be supplemented with moistening the lung and dissolving the phlegm. The prescription commonly used is:

Radix Ginseng	4-6 g
Radix Pseudostellariae	15 g
Radix Ophiopogonis	12 g
Radix Glehniae	10 g
Herba Dendrobii	10 g
Fructus Lycii	10 g
Polyporus	15 g
Poria	15 g
Bulbus Fritillariae Cirrhosae	9 g

Folium Eriobotryae 10 g
Semen Armeniace Amarum 9 g
Bulbus Lilii 10 g
Rhizoma Gynostemmatis Pentaphylli 12 g
Herba Oldenlandiae Diffusae 24 g
Radix Astragali 12 g

Add or subtract drugs according to syndrome differentiation.

3. Radiotherapy

1) Combined Therapy of TCM and Modern Medicine during Radiotherapy: The side effects of radiotherapy, include: congestion and edema of connective tissue, bronchial mucosa, atrophy of lymph follicle, subsequent acute alveolitis, which are manifested by nonproductive cough, dyspnea, irregular middle or low grade fever of short duration, small amount of hemoptysis, with moist rates in lung. If it is complicated by infection, high fever, chest pain, and aggravated dyspnea occur. After radiation pneumonitis, if atrophy of alveolar and bronchial epithelium, hyperplasia of pulmonary tissue and bronchial epithelium, occlusion of blood and lymphatic vessels and pulmonary fibrosis occur, combined therapy of TCM and moderen medicine which alleviate and prevent side effects should be implemented.

TCM treatment during radiotherapy:

Polyporus 15 g
Radix Ophiopogonis 10 g
Radix Glehniae 9 g
Rhizoma Polygonati 12 g
Fructus Lycii 12 g
Flos Lonicerae 10 g
Semen Coicis 18 g
Folium Eriobotryae 10 g
Poria 12 g
Radix Pseudostellariae 12 g
Radix Salviae Miltiorrhizae 15 g
Radix Saposhnikoviae 6 g
Bulbus Fritillariae Cirrhosae 8 g
Pumex 15 g
Radix Glycyrrhizae 4 g

Add or subtract drugs according to syndrome differentiation.

2) TCM Therapy for Treatment of Radiotherapeutic Pulmonary Fibrosis:

Radix Salviae Miltiorrhizae	15 g
Cortex Moutan	10 g
Rhizoma Chuanxiong	9 g
Radix Paeoniae Rubra	9 g
Radix Saposhnikoviae	9 g
Radix Ophiopogonis	10 g
Radix Glehniae	10 g
Radix Astragali	12 g
Polyporus	15 g
Poria	15 g
Radix Pseudostellariae	15 g
Flos Farfarae	9 g
Bulbus Fritillariae Cirrhosae	8 g
Radix Glycyrrhizae	4 g

Add or subtract drugs according to syndrome differentiation. The medicine is to be taken for 2 to 3 consecutive months or longer.

4. **Chemotherapy**

TCM therapy can be used for strengthening one's resistance and is indicated for cases of central type pulmonary carcinoma not indicated for surgery, or which have proven ioperable during exploratory thoracotomy.

PREVENTION

Publicize the knowledge of preventing cancer, improve sanitation, strengthen labor protection, give up smoking, prevent and treat chronic infection of the respiratory tract, and conduct mass general survey while pulmonary tuberculosis is being prevented and treated in order that early diagnosis and treatment may be achieved.

Chapter Seventeen
Recipes for Treating Respiratory Diseases

Asthma – relieving Decoction
(Ding chuan tang)

Ingredients

Herba Ephedrae	9 g
Semen Ginkgo	9 g
Fructus Perillae	6 g
Semen Armeniacae Amarum	9 g
Rhizoma Pinelliae	9 g
Flos Farfarae	9 g
Cortex Mori Radicis	9 g
Radix Scutellariae	6 g
Radix Glycyrrhizae	3 g

Decoct the above ingredients in a right amount of water for oral administration.

Efficacy

Facilitating the flow of the lung – qi and removing heat – phlegm to relieve asthma.

Indications

Accumulation of phlegm and heat in the lung with the attack of wind cold on the body surface marked by cough, dyspnea, profuse yellowish and viscid sputa, or accompanied by aversion to cold, fever, yellowish, greasy fur of the tongue, slippery rapid pulse.

Chronic bronchitis, bronchial asthma marked by the above – mentioned symptoms can be treated by the modified recipe.

Interpretation

Ephedra facilitates the flow of the lung - qi and disperses pathogenic factors to relieve asthma, while *Gingko - nut* astringes the lung and removes phlegm to relieve asthma. The two ingredients, one with astringing effect, and the other with the effect of dispersing, are combined to reinforce the asthma - relieving effect as well as to prevent *Ephedrae* from consuming the lung - qi. *Fructus Perillae*, *Semen Armeniacae Amarum*, *Rhizoma Pinelliae*, *Flos Farfarae* lower the adverse flow of qi and remove phlegm to relieve asthma and cough. *Mulberry bark* and *Baikal Skullcap root* clear away lung - heat to relieve cough and asthma. *Licorice root* coordinates the effects of all the other ingredients in the recipe. These drugs are combined to get the lung - qi facilitated, phlegm - heat cleared away, wind - cold pathogens expelled so that all the symptoms will disappear.

Modern researches have proved that the recipe can achieve the effects of relieving spasm of bronchial smooth muscle, expelling phlegm, arresting cough, inducing sweet and allaying fever.

Cautions

1. The recipe is contraindicated in patients with recent attack of wind - cold on the body surface without interior phlegm - heat marked by absence of sweating but asthma.

2. It is also contraindicated in patients with persistent asthma due to deficiency of qi marked by feeble pulse.

Big Blue Dragon Decoction
(Da qing long tang)

Ingredients

Herba Ephedrae	9 g
Semen Armeniacae Amarum	9 g
Radix Glycyrrhizae Praeparata	6 g
Ramulus Cinnamomi	6 g
Rhizoma Zingiberis Recens	6 g
Fructus Ziziphi Jujubae	4 pcs

Gypsum Fibrosum 30 g

Decoct the above ingredients in a right amount of water for oral administration.

Efficacy

Expelling wind - cold from the body surface and clearing away heat stagnated in the interior; mainly for cases attributive to the attack of exogenous wind - cold and stagnation of heat in the interior, which manifest as chilliness, fever, headache, general aching, anhidrosis, dyspnea, irritability, thirst, thin and white or yellowish fur on the tongue, floating and tense, rapid pulse.

Indications

1. This prescription is also used for releasing the inhibited lung - qi, and decreasing fluid - retention, promoting sweating and relieving edema, and is indicated for cases with anasarca, general aching, intolerance of cold, anhidrosis, cough, shortness of breath, fever, irritability, thin and yellow fur on the tongue, wiry and tense pulse, which are attributive to retention of cold in the superficies and heat in the interior.

2. Also applicable to cases of emphysema complicated by pulmonary infection, chronic bronchitis with acute attack, common cold, lobar pneumonia, etc. with fever and cough attributive to attack of exogenous wind - cold and retention of heat in the interior.

Interpretation

This prescription is composed by increasing the dosages of *Ephedrae* and *Glycyrrhizae* and adding *Gypsum Fibrosum*, *Zingiberis Recens* and *Ziziphi Jujubae* to the *Decoction of Ephedrae*. The dosage of *Ephedrae* is doubled and *Zingiberis Recens* is added in order to enhance the the diaphoretic effect of the *Decoction of Ephedrae*. *Gypsum Fibrosum* is used together with *Ephedrae*, *Ramulus Cinnamomi* and *Zingiberis Recens* to clear away internal heat and disperse superficial cold. *Ziziphi Jujubae* can regulate middle - jiao energy and strengthen ying and wei when it is combines with *Glycyrrhizae* and *Zingiberis Recens*, in order to promote diaphoresis without consuming yin fluid, and clear away internal heat without damaging spleen - yang.

Bolus as Kidney－yin－Tonic
(Zuo gui wan)

Ingredients

Rhizoma Rehmanniae Praeparata	240 g
Rhizoma Dioscoreae	120 g
Fructus Lycii	120 g
Fructus Corni	120 g
Radix Cyathulae	90 g
Semen Cuscutae	120 g
Colla Cornus Cervi	120 g
Colla Plastri Testudinis	120 g

Decoct the above ingredients in a right amount of water for oral administration.

Efficacy

Nourishing yin and tonifying the kidney.

Indications

Syndrome of deficiency of genuine yin marked by vertigo, lassitude in the loins and legs, seminal emission or spermatorrhea, spontaneous perspiration, night sweat, dry mouth and throat, thirst with desire for drinks, smooth tongue with little coating, and thready or rapid pulse.

Besides, syndrome of deficiency of genuine yin occurring in cases of debilitated constitution due to advanced age, chronic disorders, or recovery stage of febrile diseases can be treated with the modified recipe.

Interpretation

In the recipe, *prepared rhizome of rehmannia*, great in dosage, is used to nourish the kidney－yin; *wolfberry fruit* is to supplement the essence of life and improve acuity of vision; and *dogwood fruit* is to astringe seminal emission and sweating. Both *antler glue* and *tortoise－plastron glue*, which have close relation to health, are used in combination for replenishing and tonifying the essence, with the former tending to tonify yang and the latter tending to nourish yin. *Dodder seed* assisted by *cyathula root*, has the effect of strengthening the waist and knees and reinforcing the muscles and joints. *Chinese yam* gives the effect of nourishing and replenishing the spleen and kidney.

Directions

The boluses are made out of the powdered drugs with honey. Each bolus weighs 9 g. One bolus is to be taken each time with slightly salty liquid in the early morning and before bed time on an empty stomach.

Bolus for Invigorating Yin
(Da bu yin wan)

Ingredients

Cortex Phellodendri (fried)	15 g
*Rhizoma Anemarrhenae*9soaked with wine then fried)	15 g
Radix Rehmanniae Praeparata (steamed with wine)	30 g
Plastrum Testudinis (fried)	30 g
Pig's spinal cord	q.s.
Mel	q.s.

Decoct the above ingredients in a right amount of water for oral administration.

Efficacy

Tonifying true yin and dispersing prime – minister fire; mainly for deficiency of liver – yin and kidney – yin and flaming up of asthenic fire, manifested by hectic fever, night sweat or excessive thirst and liability to be hungry, or fever accompanied with restlessness and hemoptysis, red tongue with little fur, rapid and strong pulse at *chi* position.

Indications

1. For cases of hemoptysis, add *Cacumen Biotae* to clear away heat evil and stop bleeding; for those with profuse night sweat, add *Fructus Triticid Levis* to astringe fluid production and stop sweating.

2. The prescription may be modified for the treatment of hyperthyroidism, diabetes mellitus, consumptive diseases (e.g., pulmonary tuberculosis, tuberculosis of kidney, bone, etc.) which manifest as yin－deficiency and fire hyperactivity.

3. It should be used carefully in the cases with hypofunction of spleen and stomach manifesting anorexia and loose stools.

Interpretation

This prescription and *Bolus of Six Drugs Containing Rehmanniae Praeparata* both dealt with the disorders due to deficiency of liver－yin and kidney－yin, but the former acts more quickly and is better for the cases with stronger prime－minister fire than the latter. In the prescription, large dosage of *Rehmanniae Praeparata* and *Plastrum Testudinis* are used for tonifying the true yin to overcome the asthenic fire; *Anemarrhenae* and *Phellodendri* for clearing away prime－minister fire to preserve the true yin; *pig's spinal cord* and *honey*, substances of blood and meat, and sweet in flavor, may help to nourish the yin essence. Thus, when true yin is nourished, asthenic fire will be cleared away, and all symptoms and signs will be subsided.

Bolus of Rhei and Eupolyphaga seu Steleophaga (Dahuang zhechong wan)

Ingredients

Radix et Rhizoma Rhei (steamed)	8 g
Eupolyphaga seu Steleophaga	6 g
Radix Scutellariae	6 g
Radix Glycyrrhizae	6 g
Semen Persicae	6 g
Semen Armeniacae Amarum	6 g
Tabanus Bivittatus	6 g
Holotrichia Diomphalia	6 g
Radix Paeoniae Alba	12 g
Radix Rehmanniae	30 g
Dry Lacquer	3 g
Hirudo	8 set

Grind the above ingredients into powder and is prepared as boluses, taken with warm wine.

Efficacy

Eliminating blood stasis and masses, nourishing blood to promote tissue regeneration; mainly for consumptive diseases attributive to retention of blood stasis in the body, which are manifested by emaciation, abdominal fullness, anorexia, squamation and dryness of skin, blackish coloration around the eyes, petechiae on the tongue, wiry and unsmooth pulse, etc..

Indications

1. For cases with localized abdominal pain and tenderness, dry stools, dark purplish tongue, wiry and small, smooth pulse, which are attributive to stagnation of blood and vital energy, hyperactivity of evil and sthenia of healthy energy, the prescription may be used as an analgesic and blood－stasis eliminating agent.

2. Also indicated for cases of erysipelas of the leg with lymphangitis, dark reddish tongue, wiry and unsmooth pulse, which are attributive to obstruction of meridians by blood stasis and heat.

3. Applicable to cases of amenorrhea accompanied with localized aching and marked tenderness over the lower abdomen, emaciation, purplish spots at the margin of the tongue, wiry and small, unsmooth pulse, which are attibutive to the stagnation of liver－blood.

4. Also applicable to cases of cirrhosis of liver, pulmonary tuberculosis, gastric cancer, thrombophlebitis, osteomyelitis, etc., which are attributive to retention of blood stasis in the body or obstruction of the meridians by blood stasis and heat.

Interpretation

Rhei activates blood circulation and eliminates blood stasis; *Eupolyphaga seu Steleophaga* removes stagnated blood and eliminates masses. They act together to discharge the blood stasis with feces. № 7, 8, 11, 5 and № 12 are applied to activate blood circulation and dredge the passage of meridians, and also applied № 6 to open the stagnated lung－qi and promote blood circulation; they all serve to increase the effect of eliminating blood stasis. № 10, 9 and № 4 can nourish blood and vessels to support healthy energy. № 3 purges stagnancy – heat which may be formed by blood stasis. Wine serves to enhance the effect of other drugs.

Bupleurum and Pueraria Decoction for Dispelling Pathogens from Superficial Muscles (Chai ge jieji tang)

Ingredients

Radix Bupleuri	9 g
Radix Puerariae	9 g
Radix Scutellariae	9 g
Radix Glycyrrhizae	3 g
Radix Paeoniae	3 g
Rhizoma seu Radix Notopterygii	3 g
Radix Angelicae Dahuricae	3 g
Radix Platycodi	3 g
Gypsum Fibrosum	9 g
Rhizoma Zingiberis	3 slices
Fructus Ziziphi Jujubae	2 pieces

Decoct the above ingredients in a right amount of water for oral administration.

Efficacy

Expelling pathogenic factors from the muscles and skin and reducing fever.

Indications

Affection due to exogenous pathogenic wind – cold with heat in the interior resulting from stagnated pathogens, manifested by slight aversion to cold, high fever, headache, soreness and pain in the extremities, eye pain, dry nose, orbit pain, restlessness, insomnia, thin and yellowish coating of the tongue, and superficial and slightly full pulse.

Besides, other cases ascribed to the above syndrome such as common cold, influenza, bronchitis and toothache can be dealt with the modified recipe.

Interpretation

In the recipe, ***Bupleurum root*** and ***Pueraria root*** both possess the effect of expelling pathogenic factors from the muscles and skin and reducing fever and therefore share the role of the principal drug. № 6 and № 7, both acting as assistant drugs, are able to reinforce the action of the principal drugs in expelling pathogenic factors from the muscles and skin and is able to relieve pain. № 3 and № 9 with effect of clearing away stagnated heat exerts the role of an adjuvant drug along with № 8 used for relieving disturbances of the lung – qi to benefit in scattering and purging exopathogens and № 5 used for regulating ying and purging heat. № 10 and № 11 are capable of regulating ying and wei as well as regulating the stomach; № 4 is capable of coordinating the actions of various drugs in the recipe, acting as a guiding drug.

Cautions

1. The recipe is contraindicated in patients with symptoms of exterior wind – cold but without interior heat.
2. The recipe should not be administered for cases associated with *yangming fu* – organ disease marked by abdominal pain and constipation.

Chuanxiong Mixture
(Chuanxiong chatiao san)

Ingredients

Rhizoma Ligustici Chuanxiong	120 g
Herba Schizonepetae (remove stem)	120 g
Radix Angelicae Dahuricae	60 g
Rhizoma seu Radix Notopterygii	60 g
Radix Glycyrrhizae	60 g
Herba Asari	30 g
Radix Ledebouriellae	45 g
Herba Menthae (un – bakced)	240 g

Grind the above ingredients into fine powder, take 6 grams each time, twice a day, after mixing well with tea. It can also be decocted in water for oral administration but the dosage should be reduced proportionally on the basis of the original recipe.

Efficacy

Dispelling exopathic wind to relieve pain.

Indications

Attacks of exopathic wind marked by headache, migraine, or pain on the top of the head, aversion to cold with fever, obstruction of nose, dizziness, thin and white fur of the tongue, floating and slippery pulse.

The common cold, migraine, nervous headache, headache due to chronic rhinitis, marked by symptoms of the attack of exopathic wind can be treated by the modified recipe.

Interpretation

Chuanxiong rhizome is effective for *shaoyang* headache and *jueyin* headache (pain in the temples or pain on the top of the head), № 4, for *taiyang* headache (posterior pain of the head), № 3 for *yangming* headache (pain in the frontal bone and superciliary ridge), № 6 for *shaoyin* headache (dizziness and pain radiating to the cheeks). №8, 2 and № 7 with an elevating and dispelling effect, can be used to refresh the mind, dispel exopathic wind in assisting the principal drugs to strengthen the effect of dispelling the wind to relieve pain and induce mild diaphoresis. № 5 regulates the stomach and supplements qi, coordinates the actions of all the other drugs to prevent their excessive dispersion of qi. Taking the medicine with tea is aimed at making use of its bitter taste and cold nature to prevent the excessive warm - dryness and the excessive elevating and dispelling actions of the wind - dispelling drugs and moderate the elevating and lowering effects.

Cautions

Since it consists of more drugs with a pungent flavor which induce perspiration, the recipe is not indicated for insufficiency of qi and blood due to persistent illness or headache caused by up - stirring of liver - wind or hyperactivity of liver - yang.

Dazao Bolus of Hominis
(Da zao wan)

Ingredients

Placenta Hominis	one set
Plastrum Testudinis	60 g
Cortex Phellodendri (fried with salt)	45 g
Cortex Eucommiae	45 g
Radix Achyranthis Bidentatae	36 g
Radix Ophiopogonis	36 g
Radix Asparagi	36 g
Radix Rehmanniae	75 g
Radix Ginseng	30 g

Decoct the above ingredients in a right amount of water for oral administration.

Efficacy

Nourishing the lung and kidney, clearing away asthenic fire and lowering hectic fever due to yin – deficiency; mainly for consumptive diseases attributive to deficiency of lung – yin and kidney – yin and flaming up of asthenic fire, which manifest hectic fever, feverish sensation over the precordial region, palms and soles, nocturnal emission, night sweating, dizziness, tinnitus, lumbago, weakness of lower limbs, reddish and uncoated tongue, small and rapid pulse.

Indications

1. Applicable to cases of hemoptysis with emaciation, flushed cheeks, hectic fever, night sweating, weakness of lower extremities, uncoated and dry tongue, small and rapid, weak pulse, which are attributive to deficiency of lung – yin and kidney – yin and flaming up of asthenic fire.

2. Also indicated for cases of leucorrhagia with reddish discharge, accompanied with itching or dry and burning sensation over the pudendus, feverish sensation of precordial region, palms and soles, lumbago, tinnitus, red and uncoated tongue, small and rapid, weak pulse, which are attributive to impairment of kidney – yin and heat in the interior.

3. Also applicable to cases of hyperthyroidism, lupus erythematosus disseminatus,

dermatomyositis, pulmonary tuberculosis, bronchiectasis, etc. which are attributive to deficiency of lung-yin; and to cases of senile vaginitis and chronic cervicitis attributive to impairment of kidney-yin and interior heat resulting from yin deficiency.

Interpretation

Placenta has the effects of tonifying qi and blood, nourishing the kidney and promoting essence production, and is a principal drug for consumptive diseases. № 8, 7, 6 can nourish the lung and kidney and suppress the production of fire when the kidney-water is sufficient. Because yin-deficiency may lead to deficiency of qi, № 9 is applied to benefit qi. № 4 and № 5 are used for helping № 1 and № 8 to invigorate liver and kidney, and strengthen the tendon and bone. № 2 and № 3 used together with № 7 and № 6 have the effects of clearing away asthenic fire and lowering hectic fever.

Cinnamon Twig Decoction
(Guizhi tang)

Ingredients

Ramulus Cinnamomi	9 g
Radix Paeoniae	9 g
Radix Glycyrrhizae Praeparata	6 g
Rhizoma Zingiberis	9 g
Fructus Ziziphi Jujubae	4 pieces

Decoct the above ingredients in a right amount of water for oral administration. After taking the decoction, the patient is required to drink a small quantity of hot water or hot porridge and then lie in warm bed to induce slight perspiration.

Efficacy

Expelling pathogenic factors from the muscles and skin and regulating ying and wei to relieve exterior syndrome.

Indications

Exterior deficiency syndrome due to pathogenic wind and cold, manifested by fever, headache, perspiration with aversion to wind, nasal catarrh, retching, thin and white coating of the tongue, and floating and moderate pulse.

Equally, the recipe can be modified to deal with the common cold, influenza and others that are attributive to exterior syndrome of deficiency type caused by pathogenic wind and cold, as well as urticaria, cutaneous pruritus, eczema, neuralgia, myalgia, etc..

Interpretation

Of the ingredients in the recipe, *Cinnamon twig* is a drug with pungent, sweet and warm properties and acts as a principal drug to relieve exterior syndromes by expelling pathogenic wind and cold from the muscle and skin. № 2 is a drug with sour, bitter and slight cold properties and is used as an assistant drug for replenishing yin to astringe ying. The combination of № 1 and № 2 results in the double roles of both being diaphoretic and astringent for regulating ying and wei so as to induce sweat without impairment of yin and arrest sweat without interference in dispelling exopathogens. The are opposite and complementary to each other. № 4 can not only aid № 1 in expelling pathogenic factors from the muscles and skin but also warm the stomach and arrest vomiting. № 5 is used as tonics of stomach and blood for supplementing qi and reinforcing the middle – warmer, nourishing yin and tonifying blood; and, used in combination with № 4 as an adjuvant drug, it can regulate ying and wei. № 3 is used to tonify the middle – warmer and replenish qi and to coordinate the effect of the above drugs in the recipe.

Cautions

1. The recipe is not advisable for the exterior syndrome of excess type due to pathogenic wind and cold.

2. Patients with exterior syndrome of wind – heat type marke dby aversion to wind, perspiration as well as thirst and rapid pulse are prohibited from taking the recipe.

Decoction for Clearing Away Dryness and Treating Lung Disorders (Qing zao jiu fei tang)

Ingredients

Folium Mori	9 g
Gypsum Fibrosum (decocted first)	15 g
Radix Codonopsis Pilosulae	3 g
Semen Sesami	3 g
Colla Corii Asini	3 g
Radix Ophiopogonis	3 g
Semen Armeniacae Amarum	2 g
Radix Glycyrrhizae	2 g
Folium Eriobotryae	6 g

Decoct the above ingredients in a right amount of water for oral administration.

Efficacy

Clearing away dryness and moistening the lung; mainly for cases attributive to damage of the lung by warm – dryness, which are manifested by fever, headache, dry cough, dyspnea, dry throat and nose, vexation, thrist, dry and uncoated tongue.

Indications

1. For cases of consumptive pulmonary diseases manifested by cough with thick sputum, or dry cough with dyspnea, dry throat and thirst, emaciation, dryness of skin and hairs, red and dry tongue, small and rapid pulse, which are attributive to insufficiency of lung – yin and hyperactivity of asthenic fire, increase the dosage of *Codonopsis Pilosulae* and *Ophiopogonis* to enhance the effect of benefiting qi and pormoting the production of body fluid.

2. Applicable to cases attributive to insufficiency of lung – yin and damage of the lung by dryness – heat, which are manifested by cough with bloody sputum, dyspnea, red and uncoated tongue, weak and rapid pulse.

3. Also applicable to cases of pulmonary tuberculosis, emphysema, chronic bronchitis, atelectasis, bronchiectasis, etc. marked by dry cough or hemoptysis, which are attributive to damage of the lung by warm – dryness.

Interpretation

Mori can eliminate dryness and clear away lung - heat; *Gypsum Fibrosum* not only can discharge lung - heat but also eliminate other evils from the body surface. They increase the effect each other. № 5, 6 and № 4 can nourish yin fluid of the lung. № 3 and № 8 are applied to benefit qi and promote the production of fluid. № 7 and № 9 serve to purge lung - qi and relieve cough. As a whole, the prescription has the effects of clearing away heat and moistening dryness.

Decoction for Lifting Up Yang and Expelling Fire
(Sheng yang san huo tang)

Ingredients

Radix Puerariae	20 g
Rhizoma Cimicifugae	20 g
Radix Paeoniae Alba	12 g
Radix seu Rhizoma Notopterygii	6 g
Radix Angelicae Pubgescentis	6 g
Radix Ledebouriellae	6 g
Radix Codonopsis Pilosulae	6 g
Radix Bupleuri	6 g
Radix Glycyrrhizae	3 g
Radix Glycyrrhizae Praeparata	3 g
Rhizoma Zingiberis Recens	3 pieces
Fructus Ziziphi Jujubae	3 pieces

Decoct the above ingredients in a right amount of water for oral administration.

Efficacy

Clearing away heat and fire, lifting up yang - qi to release the depressed qi; mainly for cases attributive to dysfunction of the spleen and stagnation of heat in the stomach channel, which manifest feverish sensation of extremities and muscles, thirst, tiredness. red tongue with whitish tongue, wiry and rapid pulse.

Indications

1. Applicable to cases of leucorrhagia with whitish odorless discharge, fever, fatigue, poor appetite, loose stools, red tongue with whitish fur, slow pulse, which are attributive to hypofunction of spleen, stagnation of liver – qi and loss of essential substance.

2. Also indicated for arthralgia of heat type, manifested by pain over the joints, fever, aversion to wind, thirst, fatigue, red tongue with whitish fur, wiry and smooth pulse, which are attributive to attack of the meridians by wind and heat simultaneously, and circulatory impediment of qi and blood.

3. Also applicable to cases of influenza, poliomyelitis and functional low fever with increase of body temperature attributive to the dysfunction of spleen and stagnation of fire in the stomach meridian; to cases of endometritis and cervicitis with leucorrhagia attributive to hypofunction of spleen, stagnation of liver – qi and loss of essential substance; and to cases of rheumatic fever with arthralgia and fever attributive to simultaneous attack of wind and heat.

Interpretation

Puerariae and *Cimicifugae* can expel stomach – fire of *yangming* and also eliminate the fire stagnated in the spleen and stomach, while *Ledebouriellae* can expel the fire hidden in the spleen. *Bupleuri* and *Notopterygii* help the above drugs to lift up yang and clear away heat and fire. *Paeoniae Alba* and *Glycyrrhizae* prevent the over lifting effect of the above drugs, and lower the temperature of extremities and muscles when used together with *Angelicae Pubescentis* and *Notopterygii*. *Codonopsis Pilosulae*, *Glycyrrhizae*, *Zingiberis* and *Ziziphi Jujubae* serve to strengthen the spleen and stomach.

Decoction for Lifting Yang – qi and Benefiting Stomach (Sheng yang yi wei tang)

Ingredients

Radix Astragali seu Hedysari	12 g
Radix Codonopsis Pilosulae	10 g
Radix Paeoniae Alba	10 g
Rhizoma Atractylodis Macrocephalae	10 g

Poria	10 g
Rhizoma Pinelliae	6 g
Rhizoma et Radix Notopterygii	6 g
Radix Angelicae Pubescentis	6 g
Radix Ledebouriellae	6 g
Exocarpium Citri Grandis	6 g
Rhizoma Alismatis	6 g
Radix Bupleuri	6 g
Radix Glycyrrhizae Praeparata	3 g
Rhizoma Coptidis	3 g
Rhizoma Zingiberis Recens	5 pieces
Fructus Ziziphi Jujubae	3 pieces

Decoct the above ingredients in a right amount of water for oral administration.

Efficacy

Lifting yang – qi, invigorating the spleen, benefiting the stomach, expelling wind and dampness; mainly for cases attributive to hypofunction of the spleen and stomach and stagnation of dampness, which manifest general aching, fatigue, poor appetite, chilliness, bitter taste in the mouth, dry tongue, frequent urination, pale and corpulent tongue, white and smooth fur, slow and soft, floating pulse.

Indications

1. Indicated for cases attributive to deficiency of spleen – qi and stomachpqi and the attack of exogenous wind – dampness, which manifest as chilliness, sweating, soreness of limbs, tiredness, stuffy nose with nasal discharge, pale tongue with thin and white fur, floating and large or floating and slow pulse.

2. Applicable to cases with lienteric diarrhea, increased borborygmus, abdominal fullness, anorexia, epigastric upset after meal, spiritlessness, fatigue, pale tongue with white and smooth fur, slow and soft, floating pulse, which are attributive to hypofunction of spleen and accumulation of dampness in the stomach and intestines.

3. Also applicable to cases of pulmonary tuberculosis, chronic cholecystitis, emphysema complicated by pulmonary infection, chronic gastroenteritis, pancreatitis, irritable colon, which are attributive to hypofunction of spleen and accumulation of dampness.

Interpretation

Codonopsis Pilosulae, *Atractylodis Macrocephalae*, *Poria*, *Glycyrrhizae Praeparata*, *Citri Grandis*, *Pinelliae* and *Astragali seu Hedysari* can invigorate middle jiao, benefit vital qi, promote the function of spleen and dry dampness. In the recipe, № 2 and № 1 also have a strong effect on invigorating the lung and the spleen, and benefiting vital qi and wei – qi. № 12, 9, 7 and № 8 serve to lift up yang – qi and eliminate wind and dampness when used together with № 1. № 11 used together with № 5 can promote diuresis to relieve frequent micturition resulting from dysfunction of spleen. № 14 serves as a stomachic to improve the digestive function. № 15 and № 16 are applied for regulating ying and wei and help the above drugs to support healthy energy and eliminate evils.

Decoction for Mild Phlegm – Heat Syndrome in the Chest (Xiao xian xiong tang)

Ingredients

Rhizoma Coptidis	10 g
Rhizoma Pinelliae (washed)	10 g
Fructus Trichosanthis	25 g

Decoct the above ingredients in a right amount of water for oral administration.

Efficacy

Clearing away heat evil, eliminating phlegm, soothing the chest and dispersing stagnation; mainly for mild syndrome of phlegm – heat stagnation in the thorax, which is manifested by feeling of oppression over the chest with pain and tenderness, cough with yellow and thick sputum, and greasy fur on the tongue, floating and smooth or rapid and smooth pulse.

Indications

1. Applicable to cases with abdominal fullness, tenderness, nausea, vomiting, expectoration of yellow and thick sputum, yellow and greasy fur on the tongue, wiry and smooth pulse, which are attributive to stagnation of phlegm and heat or dampness – heat

in the middle – jiao.

2. Also applicable to cases of exudative pleuritis, bronchitis, pneumonia, et., marked by feeling of oppression over the chest and tenderness, or acute gastritis, cholecystitis, viral hepatitis, etc., marked by fullness over the epigastrium and hypochondrium and tenderness, which are attributive to the stagnation of phlegm and heat.

Decoction for Purging Lung – Heat (Xuan bai cheng qi tang)

Ingredients

Gypsum Fibrosum	20 g
Radix et Rhizoma Rhei (decoced later)	10 g
Semen Aremeniacae Amarum	8 g
Pericarpium Trichosanthis	6 g

Decoct the above ingredients in a right amount of water for oral administration.

Efficacy

Opening the stagnated lung – qi, dispersing phlegm and purging heat evil; mainly for cases attributive to heat of both the lung and the large intestine, manifested by dyspnea, profuse expectoration, constipation, hectic fever, smooth and solid pulse.

Indications

1. For cases attributive to stagnation of phlegm – heat in the lung and adverse rising of energy, which are manifested by chest pain, cough with expectoration of thick yellow sputum, bitter mouth, restlessness, yellow fur on the tongue, smooth and rapid pulse.

2. Also applicable to cases of lobar pneumonia, emphysema complicated by infection, pulmonary abscess, asthmatis bronchitis, etc. with dyspneic cough and constipation, which are attributive to heat of both the lung and the large intestine.

Decoction for Strngthening Middle Jiao and Benefiting Vital Energy (Bu zhong yi qi tang)

Ingredients

Radix Astragali seu Hedysari	15 g
Radix Codonopsis Pilosulae	15 g
Radix Angelicae Sinensis	10 g
Rhizoma Atractylodis Macrodephalae	10 g
Exocarpium Citri Grandis	6 g
Radix Glycyrrhizae Praeparata	6 g
Rhizoma Cimicifugae	3 g
Radix Bupleuri	3 g
Fructus Ziziphi Jujubae	6 g
Rhizoma Zingiberis Recens	6 g

Decoct the above ingredients in a right amount of water for oral administration.

Efficacy

Strengthening spleen, benefiting qi, lifting up yang – qi, mainly for the cases with deficiency of spleen and stomach and collapse of middle – jiao energy, manifested by shortness of breath, disinclination for speaking, tiredness, weakness, or prolapse of rectum, or fever due to deficiency of qi, pale tongue with white fur, empty and weak pulse.

Indications

1. This prescription is originally applied to fever due to internal damage, and now commonly for prolapse of rectum, gastroptosis and prolapse of uterus due to deficiency and collapse of qi.

2. Applicable to cases of common cold with deficiency of qi manifesting lingering fever, profuse sweating, pale tongue and weak pulse.

3. Also applicable to cases of septicemia, pulmonary tuberculosis, aplastic anemia, leukemia and summer fever which are manifested by fever due to deficiency of qi.

Interpretation

Astragali seu Hedysari has the effects of tonifying and lifting up qi; № 2, 4 and № 6 have the effects of strengthening the spleen and regulating the stomach, helping № 1 to tonify qi. While № 7 and № 8 have the effects of leading the stomach – qi upward, helping № 1 to lift up qi. № 3 can nourish blood and help qi to flow toward its bases. The case with deficiency of qi usually suffers from stagnation of qi, so the prescription includes № 5, 10 and № 9 to regulate qi and the stomach.

Decoction of Adenophorae Strictae and Ophiopogonis (Shashen maidong tang)

Ingredients

Radix Adenophorae	15 g
Radix Ophiopogonis	15 g
Rhizoma Polygonati Odorati	10 g
Semen Dolichoris	10 g
Radix Trichosanthis	10 g
Folium Mori	5 g
Radix Glycyrrhizae	3 g

Decoct the above ingredients in a right amount of water for oral administration.

Efficacy

Nourishing the lung and stomach, promoting the production of fluid, moistening the dryness evil; mainly for cases attributive to damage of the lung and stomach by dryness and consumption of body fluid, which are manifested by dry cough, dry throat, thirst, red uncoated tongue, small and rapid pulse.

Indications

1. Applicable to cases of diabetes involving the upper jiao manifested by polydipsia, dry mouth and tongue, polyuria, red uncoated tongue, small and rapid pulse, which are attributive to insufficiency of lung – yin and failuree of lung – fluid distribution.

2. For cases of hemoptysis accompanied with irritability, feverish face, dry throat, red uncoated tongue, small and rapid pulse, which are attributive to deficiency of both lung－yin and kidney－yin and flaming up of asthenic fire, add *Cacumen Biotae* and *Colla Corii Asini* to cool the blood and stop bleeding.

3. Also applicable to cases of chronic pharyngitis, chronic laryngitis, tuberculosis of pharynx and larynx, pulmonary tuberculosis, silicosis, etc. marked by dry cough jor hemoptysis, or cases of hyperthyroidism, thyroiditis, diabetes mellitus, etc. marked by polydipsia, which are attributive to insufficiency of lung－yin.

Interpretation

Adenophorae Strictae, *Ophiopogonis*, *Polygonati Odorati* and *Trichosanthis* are applied for nourishing yin－fluid of lung and stomach, and clearing away dryness－heat from the lung and stomach. *Mori* has the effects of releasing the stagnated lung－qi and relieving cough. *Dolichoris* used together with *Glycyrrhizae* serves to nourish stomach－qi and promote the function of spleen and stomach, and to provide fluid to the lung.

Decoction of Arctii for Soothing Muscles (Niubang jieji tang)

Ingredients

Fructus Arctii	12 g
Fructus Forsythiae	12 g
Radix Scrophulariae	12 g
Fructus Gardeniae	10 g
Cortex Moutan Radicis	10 g
Spica Prunellae	10 g
Herba Dendrobii	10 g
Herba Schizonepetae	6 g
Herba Menthae	3 g

Decoct the above ingredients in a right amount of water for oral administration.

Efficacy

Clearing away heat and toxic material, expelling wind from the body surface and reducing swelling; mainly for skin infection of the head and neck, accompanied with fever, chilliness, headache, dry mouth, oliguria with reddish urine, red tongue with yellow fur, smooth and rapid pulse, which are attributive to the attack of wind, fire, toxic material and heat.

Indications

1. Applicable to cases of common cold attributive to attack of exogenous wind－heat, which manifest as fever, chilliness, headache, sore－throat, thirst, thinyellow fur on the tongue, floating and rapid pulse.

2. For cases of measles with interrupted eruption, fever, chilliness, sneezing, cough, congestion of conjunctiva, lacrimation, thirst, red tongue with thin yellow fur, floating and rapid pulse, which are attributive to attack of heat and toxic material to the lung and stomach, and retention of the pathogens in the superficies.

3. Also to cases of hordeolum accompanied with fever, chilliness, headache, thirst, red tongue and rapid pulse, which are attributive to attack of heat and toxic material to the eyes.

4. For cases of upper respiratory viral infection and iffluenza attributive to the attack of exogenous wind－heat; and for cases of chalazion and tarsitis attributive to the attack of heat evil and toxic material attack to the eyes.

Decoction of Astragali seu Hedysari for Warming Middle Jiao (Huangqi jianzhong tang)

Ingredients

Ramulus Cinnamomi	10 g
Rhizoma Zingiberis Recens	10 g
Radix Paeoniae Alba	20 g
Radix Astragali seu Hedysari	15 g
Radix Glycyrrhizae Praeparata	6 g
Saccharum Granorum	30 g

Fructus Ziziphi Jujubae 7 pieces

Decoct the above ingredients in a right amount of water for oral administration.

Efficacy

Warming middle jiao, tonifying, alleviating pain, harmonizing yin and yang, and regulating ying and wei.

Indications

1. To cases of fever attributive to deficiency of spleen and stomach－qi, and floating up of yang－qi, which manifest as increase of body temperature with preference for hot drink, aversion to cold, cold limbs, sweating, shortness of breath, fatigue, poor appetite, pale tongue with white fur, floating and large weak pulse.

2. For cases of jaundice attributive to hypofunction of spleen, decreased production of qi and blood, and failure of nourishing skin and muscles, which manifest as yellowish coloration, dryness and lusterless appearance of the skin, shortness of breath, fatigue, polyuria with clear urine, pale and swelling tongue, white and smooth fur, slow pulse.

3. To cases of gastroptosis, peptic ulcer, prolapse of gastric mucosa, leukemia, aplastic anemia, pulmonary tuberculosis, hemolytic jaundice, ancylostomiasis, etc. attributive to hypofunction of spleen.

Decoction of Belamcandae and Ephedrae
(Shegan mahuang tang)

Ingredients

Rhizoma Belamcandae 9 g
Herba Ephedrae 9 g
Radix Asteris 9 g
Flos Farfarae 9 g
Rhizoma Pinelliae Praeparata 9 g
Rhizoma Zingiberis Recens 12 g
Fructus Schisandrae 6 g
Herba Asari 3 g

Fructus Ziziphi Jujubae	3 pieces

Decoct the above ingredients in a right amount of water for oral administration.

Efficacy

Warming the lung to disperse phlegm, relieving cough and dyspnea.

Indications

1. To serious cases of whooping cough with white and greasy fur on the tongue, wiry and smooth pulse, which are attributive to the retention of phlegm in the lung and failure of lung-qi to be clear and descendant.

2. For cases with retention of cold-phlegm in the interior but without the attack of exogenous evil.

3. To cases of bronchial asthma, asthmatic bronchitis, chronic bronchitis, adenovirus pneumonia, eosinophilia, etc., marked by cough and dyspnea, which are attributive to retention of cold-phlegm in the lung and adverse rising of lung-qi.

Decoction of Cinnamomi and Aconiti (Guizhi fuzi tang)

Ingredients

Ramulus Cinnamomi	12 g
Radix Aconiti Praeparata	10 g
Rhizoma Zingiberis Recens	10 g
Fructus Ziziphi Jujubae	8 pcs
Radix Glycyrrhizae Praeparata	6 g

Decoct the above ingredients in a right amount of water for oral administration.

Efficacy

Expelling wind and dampness, warming meridians and eliminating cold.

Indications

1. To cases with yang - deficiency constitution and affection of wind - cold, which manifest as chilliness, fever, aversion to wind, sweating, headache, cold limbs, tiredness, somnolence, white and greasy fur on the tongue, sunken and slow pulse.

2. For cases with chest pain referring to the back, feeling of oppression over the chest, tiredness, white and greasy fur on the tongue, wiry and slow pulse, which are attributive to accumulation of cold - dampness.

3. To cases of rheumatic arthritis, sciatica periarthritis, etc. with chilliness and fever attributive to yang - deficiency and affection of exogenous wind - cold; and to cases of emphysema, coronary heart disease, rheumatic heart disease, etc. with chest pain attributive to accumulation of wind - phlegm.

Decoction of Codonopsis Pilosulae and Perillae (Shen su yin)

Ingredients

Folium Perillae	12 g
Radix Codonopsis Pilosulae	10 g
Radix Puerariae	10 g
Radix Peucedani	10 g
Rhizoma Pinelliae	10 g
Poria	10 g
Fructus Aurantii	10 g
Exocarpium Citri Grandis	6 g
Radix Glycyrrhizae	6 g
Radix Platycodi	6 g
Radix Aucklandiae	3 g
Rhizoma Zingiberis Recens	3 pcs
Fructus Ziziphi Jujubae	3 pcs

Decoct the above ingredients in a right amount of water for oral administration.

Efficacy

Benefiting and regulating qi, expelling the evils from the body surface and eliminating sputum.

Indications

1. For cases accompanied with vomiting, omit *Glycyrrhizae* and *Platycodi* and add *Herba Agastachis*, or *Caulis Perillae* to eliminate dampness; for cases accompanied with discharge of loose stools, omit *Glycyrrhizae* and *Platycodi*, and add *Atractylodis* to activate the spleen and dry the dampness.

2. To cases of common cold of gastrointestinal type complicated by infection, which are attributive to affection of wind－cold evil in cases of deficiency of qi.

Decoction of Colla Corii Asini for Invigorating Lung
(Bufei e'jiao tang)

Ingredients

Colla Corii Asini	12 g
Fructus Aristolochiae	12 g
Fructus Arctii	10 g
Semen Armeniacae Amarum	10 g
Radix Glycyrrhizae	3 g
Semen Oryzae Glutinosae	15 g

Decoct the above ingredients in a right amount of water for oral administration.

Efficacy

Nourishing yin, invigorating lung, clearing away lung－heat and relieving cough.

Indications

1. To cases of hemoptysis with discharge of fresh blood, dry throat, dry stool, flushed cheeks, night sweat, red and uncoated tongue, small and rapid pulse, which are

attributive to yin – deficiency and fire hyperactivity causing damage of yang – collaterals.

2. For cases of prolonged aphonia accompanied with dry throat, sore – throat, dry cough, red and uncoated tongue, small and rapid pulse, which are attributive to damage of the lung by dryness – heat and hyperactivity of asthenic fire.

3. To chronic bronchitis, emphysema, pulmonary tuberculosis, etc. marked by cough or hemoptysis, which are attributive to deficiency of lung – yin; or cases of chronic laryngitis, polypus of vocal cord, tec. marked by aphonia, which are attributive to damage of the lung by drness – heat and hyperactivity of asthenic fire.

Decoction of Coptidis for Detoxification
(Neishu huanglian tang)

Ingredients

Rhizoma Coptidis	9 g
Radix Scutellariae	9 g
Fructus Gardeniae	9 g
Fructus Forsythiae	9 g
Radix Angelicae Sinensis	9 g
Radix Paeoniae Alba	9 g
Radix Aucklandiae	6 g
Herba Menthae	3 g
Radix Platycodi	3 g
Radix Glycyrrhizae	3 g
Radix et Rhizoma Rhei	6 g

Decoct the above ingredients in a right amount of water for oral administration.

Efficacy

Clearing away heat and toxic material, activating blood circulation, relieving swelling and promoting bowel movement.

Indications

To cases of jaundice manifested by bright yellow coloration over the body, fever, thirst, oliguria, reddish urine, constipation, yellow and greasy fur on the tongue, wiry and rapid pulse, which are attributive to the accumulation of dampness – heat.

To cases of appendicitis, liver abscess and lung abscess, to cases of cellulitis, lymphadenitis and mastitis and to cases of acute cholecystitis, icterus infectious hepatitis and cholelithiasis with jaundice attributive to the attack of dampness – heat.

Decoction of Ephedrae, Armeniacae Amarum, Coicis and Glycyrrhizae (Ma xing yi gan tang)

Ingredients

Herba Ephedrae	6 g
Radix Glycyrrhizae Praeparata	6 g
Semen Armeniacae Amarum	9 g
Semen Coicis	30 g

Decoct the above ingredients in a right amount of water for oral administration.

Efficacy

Expelling wind and dampness and alleviating pain, mainly for cases attributive to retention of wind – dampness in the superficies, which manifest as general aching, fever which is higher in the afternoon, thirst but refusing to drink, thin and white fur on the tongue, floating and rapid pulse.

Indications

1. To edema of wind origin manifested by general anasarca beginning from the eyes, artharalgia, chilliness, fever, cough, shortness of breath, thin and white fur on the tongue, floating and rapid pulse, which is attributive to attack of wind and water in the muscle and skin.

2. For cases attributive to attack of wind during sweating with affection of dampness resulting in stagnation of ying – qi, which manifest as urticaria, aversion to cold, fever, thin and white fur on the tongue, floating and rapid pulse, add *Periostracum Cicadae* to the prescription.

3. To cases of acute rheumatic arthritis and influenza, with general aching and fever attributive to attack of wind – dampness evil to the superficies; to cases of acute nephritis and edema of pregnancy with puffiness of eyes and fever attributive to attack of wind and water; and to cases of dermatitis medicamentosa attributive to attack of wind and dampness and the stagnation of ying – qi.

Interpretation

Ephedrae can dispel wind – dampness through its diaphoretic effect. Armeniacae Amarum has the effect of releasing the inhibited lung – qi, which can help *Ephedrae* to disperse the superficial wind – dampness. *Coicis* can clear away dampness and heat, activate the joints and relieve muscular spasms. It can relieve pain when it combines with *Ephedrae*. *Glycyrrhizae* can decrease the diaphoretic effect of *Ephedrae* and increase the analgesic effect of *Coicis*.

Decoction of Ephedrae, Armeniacae Amarum, Glycyrrhizae and Gypsum Fibrosum (Ma xing shi gan tang)

Ingredients

Herba Ephedrae	10 g
Radix Glycyrrhizae Praeparata	6 g
Semen Armeniacae Amarum	10 g
Gypsum Fibrosum	30 g

Decoct the above ingredients in a right amount of water for oral administration.

Efficacy

Releasing the inhibited lung – qi, purging heat evil, relieving asthma and cough.

Indications

To cases with and without sweating. For cases of asthma without sweating attributive to stagnation of heat evil in the lung, the dosage of *Gypsum Fibrosum* applieed should be triple than that of *Ephedrae*. For cases of asthma with sweating attributive to severe lung－heat, the dosage of *Gypsum Fibrosum* should be five times more than that of *Ephedrae*.

2. For cases of measles, no matter the eruption is complete or incomplete, which are accompanied with fever, dyspnea and movement of ala nasi, indicating the retention of toxic material and extreme lung－heat, add *Radix Arnebiae seu Lithospermi* and *Stigma Crocus* to eliminate toxic material and let out the skin eruptions.

3. To cases of acute bronchitis, bronchopneumonia, lobar pneumonia and measles complicated by pneumonia, which are attributive to stagnation of heat evil in the lung.

Interpretation

Gypsum Fibrosum not only can clear away lung－heat but also can let out evil－heat, and serves to get rid of the source of evil－heat. *Ephedrae* has the effects of releasing the inhibited lung－qi, and its diaphoretic effect is diminished when it is used together with *Gypsum Fibrosum*. It serves to open a breath for the stagnated heat. These two drugs inhibit each other. The prescription exerts an acrid－cold action for releasing the inhibited lung－qi and letting out heat evil. *Armeniacae Amarum* possesses a descending action, which help *Ephedrae* to relieve asthma and cough. *Glycyrrhizae Praeparata* has the effects of regulating the middle jiao and protecting the stomach.

Decoction of Ephedrae, Asari and Aconiti (Mahuang xixin fuzi tang)

Ingredients

Herba Ephedrae	6 g
Herba Asari	3 g
Radix Aconiti Praeparata	10 g

Decoct the above ingredients in a right amount of water for oral administration.

Efficacy

Strengthening yang to expel the superficial evils.

Indications

1. For affection of exogenous evil in the cases with yang – deficiency which is not so severe. Attention should be paid to that when the yang – qi is much weakened and watery diarrhea ensues, diaphoretics may cause exhaustion of yang – energy.

2. To cases of emphysema complicated by infection, acute exacerbation of chronic nephritis, etc. manifested by chilliness, shortness of breath or edema, which are attributive to yang – deficiency complicated by the attack of wind – cold evil.

Decoction of Gardeniae and Sojae Praeparatum (Zhi zi chi tang)

Ingredients

Fructus Gardeniae 10 g
Semen Sojae Praeparatum 12 g

Decoct the above ingredients in a right amount of water for oral administration.

Efficacy

Dischagrging the stagnated heat and relieving irritability.

Indications

1. For cases manifest as fever, irritability, insomnia, feeling of oppresion over the chest and epigastrium, red tongue with yelllowish fur, rapid pulse. For cases mentioned above accompanied with vomiting which is resulting from damage of the stomach by erroneous application of purgative or emetic. For those accompanied with feeling of fullness over the chest and abdomen resulting from damage of the spleen by erroneous application of purgative.

2. To cases of jaundice with bright yellow coloration of the skin, fever, thirst, irritability, oliguria with yellow urine, or constipation, yellow and smooth fur on the tongue, wiry and rapid pulse, which are attributive to attack of dampness – heat to the liver and gallbladder.

3. To cases of upper respiratory infection, esophagitis, vegetative nervous disorder

and chronic gastritis with fever and irritability, which are attributive to the stagnation of heat in the chest; to cases of acute iterus infectious hepatitis and cholecystitis with jaundice attributive to the attack of dampness – heat; and to cases of chronic rhinitis, epidemic hemorrhagic fever, which are attributive to the stagnation of heat in the lung.

Deccotion of Ginseng for Nourishing Qi and Ying
(Renshen yang rong tang)

Ingredients

Radix Paeoniae Alba	15 g
Radix Rehmanniae Praeparata	15 g
Radix Codonopsis Pilosulae	10 g
Radix Astragali seu Hedysari	10 g
Rhizoma Atractylodis Macrocephalae	10 g
Poria	10 g
Radix Angelicae Sinensis	10 g
Exocarpium Citri Grandis	6 g
Fructus Schisandrae	6 g
Radix Glycyrrhizae Praeparata	3 g
Cortex Cinnamomi	3 g
Radix Polygalae	3 g
Rhizoma Zingiberis Recens	3 pcs
Fructus Ziziphi Jujubae	3 pcs

Decoct the above ingredients in a right amount of water for oral administration.

Efficacy

Benefiting qi, tonifying blood, strengthening spleen and nourishing heart; mainly for consumptive diseases manifested by palpitation, amnesia, insomnia, dreaminess, tiredness, profuse sweating, poor appetite, shortness of breath, dyspnea upon exertion, pale tongue, sunken and weak pulse, which are attributive to insufficiency of qi and blood, and hypofunction of heart and spleen.

Indications

Applicable to cases of irregular (or delayed) menstruation with scanty pale discharge, sallow complexion, palpitation, dizziness, shortness of breath, fatigue, poor appetite, pale tongue, which are attributive to deficiency of liver – blood and spleen – qi and failure of releasing stagnated qi and controlling blood.

2. Also indicated for the late stage of pyogenic infection of skin when the acute inlammation subsides but the qi and blood are deficient, which manifest lesion with discharge of thin purulent fluid, dark greyish coloration but without granulation, and accompanied with lusterless complexion and pale tongue.

3. Also applicable to cases of pulmonary tuberculosis, rheumatic heart diseases, gastric ulcer, tuberculous abscess, carbuncle, phlebeurysma of the lower limbs, etc. which are attributive to deficiency of qi and blood.

Interpretation

The prescription is composed by omitting *Rhizoma Ligustici Chuanxiong* and adding *Astragali seu Hedysari*, *Cortex Cinnamomi*, *Citri Grandis*, *Schisandrae* and *Polygalae* to the *Decoction of Eight Ingredients for Tonifying Qi and Blood*. *Ligustici Chuanxiong* is omitted because the effect of activating blood circulation is not desired. The effect of tonifying blood and promoting blood production is obtained when *Astragali seu Hedysari* is used together with *Angelicae Sinensis*. *Cortex Cinnamomi* used together with *Zingiberis Recens*, *Ziziphi Jujubae* can accelerate the growth of qi and blood. *Polygalae* and *Schisandrae* adding to *Codonopsis Pilosulae* and *Astragali seu Hedysari* serve to benefit the heart – qi and tranquilizing. *Citri Grandis* is used for regulating qi and stomach to decrease the indigestibility of the tonics.

Decoction of Glycyrrhizae and Zingiberis
(Gancao ganjiang tang)

Ingredients

Radix Glycyrrhizae Praeparata 12 g
Rhizoma Zingiberis 10 g

Decoct the above ingredients in a right amount of water for oral administration.

Efficacy

Strengthening spleen - yang; mainly for cases attributive to deficiency of spleen - yang and stomach - yang, which manifest chilliness, spontaneous sweating, cold limbs, flat taste in the mouth, no thirst, pale tongue with white and smooth fur, slow pulse.

Indications

1. For cases of hematemesis with pale complexion, profuse sweating over the head, cold breathing, cold limbs, slow pulse, which are attributive to the deficiency - cold of spleen and stomach and failure of keeping the blood inside the vessels, roasted *ginger* is used instead of dried *ginger* to enhance the effect of warming middle jiao and stopping bleeding.

2. Applicable to cases with abdominal pain which can be alleviated by warmth and aggravated by coldness, increased secretion of saliva, discharge of watery urine, white and smooth fur on the tongue, wiry and tense pulse, which are attributive to involvement of yang during exogenous febrile disease.

3. Also indicated for consumptive pulmonary diseases manifested by cough with foamy expectoration, no thirst, dizziness, chilliness, pale tongue with white fur, slow pulse, which are attributive to the yang - deficiency of upper - jiao and asthenia - cold of lung - qi.

4. Also applicable to cases of peptic ulcer, chronic gastritis, prolapse of gastric mucosa, etc. marked by cold limbs, sweating, or hematemesis, or abdominal pain, which are attributive to deficiency of spleen - yang and stomach - yang; and to cases of chronic obstructive emphysema and pulmonary abscess attributive to asthenia - cold of lung - qi.

Interpretation

Glycyrrhizae has the effect of benefiting middle - jiao energy, and *Zingiberis* serves to warm the middle - jiao and expel cold. The two drugs used together can strengthen spleen - yang to eliminate cold.

Decoction of Gypsum Fibrosum and Three Yellows
(Sanhuang shigao tang)

Ingredients

Gypsum Fibrosum (decocted first 30 g

Radix Scutellariae	10 g
Rhizoma Coptidis	10 g
Cortex Phellodendri	10 g
Fructus Gardeniae	10 g
Semen Sojae Praeparatum	10 g
Herba Ephedrae	3 g
Rhizoma Zingiberis Recens	3 pcs
Fructus Ziziphi Jujubae	2 pcs
Folium Camelliae Sinensis	6 g

Decoct the above ingredients in a right amount of water for oral administration.

Efficacy

Expelling the pathogens from both the interior and the superficies, purging fire and eliminating toxic materials; mainly for seasonal febrile diseases involving both the interior and superficies, which manifest as high fever, chilliness, anhidrosis, flushed cheeks, dryness of teeth and nose, extreme thirst, severe headache, irritability or even mania, red tongue with yellow fur, bounding and rapid or smooth and rapid pulse.

Indications

1. For cases with yang macules which are punctate or pieces and bright red in colour, accompanied with high fever, thirst, flushed cheeks, conjunctival congestion, red or crimson tongue with yellow fur, bounding and rapid pulse, which are attributive to stagnation of heat in the *yangming* channel involving *yingfen* and *xuefen*, use *Radix Rehmanniae* instead of *Ephedrae* and *Sojae Praeparatum*.

2. Also applicable to cases suffering from common cold, encephalitis B, typhoid fever and paratyphoid fever with high fever, which are attributive to attack of potent heat to both interior and the superficies; and to cases of epidemic hemorrhagic fever, typhus fever, which are attributive to the stagnation of heat in the *yangming* channel involving *yingfen* and *xuefen*.

3. Applicable to infections of skin and subcutaneous tissues acccompanied with high fever, irritability, extreme thirst, oliguria with reddish urine, red tongue with yellow fur, wiry and rapid pulse, which are attributive to retnetion of heat and toxic material in the superficies when the pathogens are potent and the healthy energy is still strong.

Interpretation

Gypsum Fibrosum can clear away the interior heat and acts as the chief drug of the prescription. *Ephedrae* and *Sojae Praeparatum* are applied to promote sweating and discharge the heat outside. The above three durgs used together can expel heat from both the interior and the superficies. Since there is a large amount of heat in the triple－jiao, *Scutellariae* is applied to clear away the heat in the upper－jiao. *Gardeniae* and *Camelliae Sinensis* can discharge the heat of triple－jiao from the urine. *Zingiberis* and *Ziziphi Jujubae* serve to regulate *ying* and *wei*.

Decoction of Larger Dosage of Pinelliae
(Da banxia tang)

Ingredients

Rhizoma Pinelliae (washed)	12 g
Radix Codonopsis Pilosulae	10 g
Mel (mixed with the decoction)	20 g

Decoct the above ingredients in a right amount of water for oral administration.

Efficacy

Decreasing fluid retention, dispersing the stagnation, lowering the abnormla rising qi, stopping vomiting, benefiting qi and moistening dryness; mainly for cases attributive to hypofunction of stomach with fluid retention and damage of yin, which manifest as vomiting long after meal, constipation, reddish dry tongue, soft and floating pulse.

Indications

1. For cases attributive to insufficiency of yin and qi and decresed production of body fluid, which manifest as cough with expectoration of thick and foamy sputum, thirst, dry throat, dizziness, shortness of breath, reddish tongue, small and rapid pulse, the dosage of *Codonopsis Pilosulae* may be increased to 15 g, while *Pinelliae* maintained in the original dose.

2. Also applicable to cases of volvulus of stomach cardiospasm, pylorochesis, etc. with vomiting attributive to hypofunction of stomach with fluid retention and damage of

yin; and to cases of chronic bronchitis, pulmonary tuberculosis, pleurisy, etc. attributive to insufficiency of yin and qi, and decreased production of body fluid.

Interpretation

Pinelliae can dry the dampness and decrease fluid retention, and also lower the abnormal rising qi to stop vomiting. *Codonopsis Pilosulae* can strengthen the spleen and calm the stomach, and its indigestive effect will be counteracted by *Pinelliae*. Aiming at the presence of yin damage resulting from prolonged vomiting, *Mel* is applied for nourishing the spleen and stomach and moistening the intestines, and also for decreasing the toxicity of *Pinelliae*. In turn, the emetic of honey may be inhibited by *Pinelliae*.

Decoction of Lilli for Strengthening Lung (Baihe gujin tang)

Ingredients

Radix Rehmanniae (crude)	12 g
Radix Rehmanniae Praeparata	18 g
Radix Ophiopogonis	10 g
Bulbus Lilli	10 g
Radix Paeoniae Alba	6 g
Radix Angelicae Sinensis	6 g
Bulbus Fritillariae Cirrhosae	6 g
Radix Scrophulariae	6 g
Radix Glycyrrhizae	3 g
Radix Platycodi	3 g

Decoct the above ingredients in a right amount of water for oral administration.

Efficacy

Nourishing the lung and kidney, moisturizing the lung and dispersing phlegm; mainly for cases attributive to deficiency of lung – yin and kidney – yin and consumption of the lung by asthenic fire, which are manifested by cough, dryness of the throat, sorethroat, shortness of breath, bloody sputum, feverish sensation of palms and soles, red uncoated tongue, small and rapid pulse.

Indications

1. For cases of pulmonary tuberculosis manifested by hectic fever, night sweat, flushed cheeks, irritability, insomnia, dry cough, shortness of breath, nocturnal emission, fatigue, red uncoated tongue, small and rapid pulse, which are attributive to consumption of lung – yin with fatigue of nourishing the kidney, add *Carapax Trionycis*.

2. Applicable to cases of aphonia accompanied with dry throat, dry cough, restlessness, insomnia, feverish sensation of palms, soles and precordial region, tinnitus, dizziness, lassitude of the loins and joints, red uncoated tongue, small and rapid pulse, which are attributive to deficiency of lung – yin and kidney – yin.

3. Also applicable to cases of chronic pharyngitis, bronchitis, bronchiectasis, pulmonary tuberculosis, polypus of vocal cord, carcinoma of larynx, etc., which are attributive to deficiency of lung – yin and kidney – yin, and damage of the lung by asthenic fire.

Interpretation

Lilli moisturizes the lung and relieves cough, and helps *Ophiopogonis* to nourish lung fluid. *Radix Rehmanniae Praeparata* accompanied with *Scrophulariae* serve to nourish kidney – yin and inhibit fire so as to relieve cough. *Fritillariae Cirrhosae*, *Platycodi* and *Glycyrrhizae* can promote sputum discharge and relieve cough. *Rehmanniae*, *Angelicae Sinensis* and *Paeoniae Alba* nourish blood and regulate yin, and enhance the effect of *Lilli* and *Rehmanniae Praeparata*. In sum the prescription serves to promote the production of yin – fluid to nourish the lung and kidney, and to suppress asthenic fire and relieve the symptoms.

Decoction of Mori and Armeniacae Amarum

Ingredients

Folium Mori	6 g
Bulbus Fritillariae Thunbergii	6 g
Semen Sojae Praeparatum	6 g
Fructus Gardeniae	6 g
Exocarpium Pyrus	6 g
Semen Armeniacae Amarum	9 g
Radix Adenophorae Strictae	12 g

Decoct the above ingredients in a right amount of water for oral administration.

Efficacy

Moistening the lung and promoting the production of fluid; mainly for affection of exogenous warm – dryness, manifested by fever, headache, dry cough, thirst, red tongue with thin, white and dry fur, floating and rapid pulse.

Indications

1. For cases with sorethroat, add *Fructus Arctii* to soothe the throat; for cases with expectoration of yellow and thick sputum, add *Fructus Aristolochiae* and *Pericarpium Trichosanthis* to clear away heat and disperse sputum.

2. For cases of hemoptysis attributive to damage of the lung by wind – heat, manifested by itching over the throat, cough with fresh bloody sputum, dry mouth and nose, fever, red tongue with thin and yellow fur, floating and rapid pulse, omit *Sojae Praeparatum* and add *Rhizoma Imperatae* to clear away heat and cool the blood.

3. Applicable to cases of measles during the disappearance of rashes, manifested by dryness of skin, nose and throat, low fever, thirst, dry cough, thin white and dry fur on the tongue.

4. Also applicable to cases of common cold, chronic bronchitis, pulmonary tuberculosis, pleurisy, etc. with dry cough attributive to affection of exogenous warm – dryness.

Interpretation

Mori is good for clearing away wind – heat or dry – heat in the lung channel and the body surface, but its effect is not strong enough, so it is assisted by *Gardeniae* and *Sojae Praeparatum* to clear away lung – heat and dryness. *Armeniacae Amarum* can release the stagnated lung – qi; *Fritillariae Thunbergii* is good for dispersing dry sputum; *Adenophorae Strictae* and *Exocarpium Pyrus* can produce fluid and disperse sputum. The above four drugs used together exert antitussive, expectorant, fluid producing and lung – qi releasing effects.

Decoction of Mulberry Leaf and Chrysanthemum (Sang ju yin)

Ingredients

Folium Mori	7.5 g
Flos Chrysanthemi	3 g
Semen Armeniacae Amarum	6 g
Fructus Forsythiae	5 g
Herba Menthae	2.5 g
Radix Platycodi	6 g
Radix Glycyrrhizae	2.5 g
Rhizoma Phragmitis	6 g

Decoct the above ingredients in a right amount of water for oral administration.

Efficacy

Relieving the exterior syndrome with drugs pungent in flavor and cool in property, facilitating the flow of the lung – qi to relieve cough.

Indications

The onset of cough due to wind – heat, marked by cough, mild feverish body, slight thirst, thin and white coating of the tongue and floating pulse.

The modification of the above recipe can be adopted for the treatment of such diseases as common cold, influenza, acute bronchitis, bronchial pneumonia and acute tonsillitis that indicate the exterior syndrome due to wind – heat.

Interpretation

Among the drugs of the recipe, *Mulberry leaf* and *Chrysanthemum flower* sweet in flavor and cool in property with mild effect, act in combination as principal drugs for expelling pathogenic heat from the lung and wei system to relieve cough. *Peppermint* with the effect of dispelling wind – heat acts as an assistant drug together with *Bitter apricot kernel* and *Platycodon root* to promote the dispersing function of the lung to relieve cough. *Forsythia fruit*, pungent and bitter in flavor and cold in property, possesses the effect of dispersing wind – heat from exterior and is used as an adjuvant drug with *Reed rhizome* which is sweet in flavor and cold in property and has the effect of clearing away heat, and promoting the production of body fluid to quench thirst. *Licorice root* is used as a mediator for coordinating various effects of the drugs in the recipe.

Clinically and experimentally, it is ascertained that the above recipe has the functions of relieving cough, removing phlegm, resisting bacteria, subduing inflammation as well as inducing mild sweat and allaying fever.

Cautions

1. Those with cough due to exogenous wind – cold are prohibited from taking this recipe.

2. Since the drugs in the recipe are of dispersing effect, they should not be decocted for a long time.

Decoction of Notopterygium for Rheumatism (Qianghuo shengshi tang)

Ingredients

Rhizoma seu Radix Notopterygii	6 g
Radix Angelicae Pubescentis	6 g
Rhizoma Ligustici	3 g
Radix Ledebouriellae	3 g
Radix Glycyrrhizae Praeparata	3 g
Rhizoma Ligustici Chuanxiong	3 g
Fructus Vitici	2 g

Decoct the above ingredients in a right amount of water for oral administration.

Efficacy

Expeling wind – dampness, arresting pain and relieving the exterior syndrome.

Indications

Attack of wind – damp on the body surface marked by heavy sensation and pain of the head and body or general aching and difficulty in turning round or sidewards, slight aversion to wind and cold, white fur of the tongue and floating and slow pulse.

The common cold, influenza, sciatica and chronic rheumatic arthritis ascribed to the syndrome of attack of wind – damp on the body surface can be treated by the modified recipe.

Interpretation

Both as principal drugs, ***Notopterygium root*** can dispel wind－dampness from the upper part of the body and ***Pubescent angelica root*** tends to dispel wind－dampness from the lower part. The combined use of the two can expel wind－dampness from the whole body and the joints to treat arthralgia. ***Ledebouriella root*** and ***Ligusticum root***, as assistant drugs, can dispel wind－cold to relieve headache. ***Chuanxiong rhizome*** promotes blood circulation and expels wind to arrest pain and ***Chastetree fruit*** dispels wind to arrest pain, both acting as adjuvant drugs. ***Prepared licorice root***, as a guiding drug, coordinates the effects of the other drugs in the recipe.

Modern researches have proved that the recipe has great effect of relieving pain and is effective in inducing diaphoresis, promoting blood circulation, resisting viruses and inducing diuresis.

Cautions

Since the recipe is one for relieving the exterior syndrome by dispelling wind and dampness with drugs pungent in flavor and warm in nature, it is contraindicated in patients with wind－heat syndrome due to invasion of exopeathogen or those suffering from the common cold with perspiration.

Decoction of Ophiopogonis
(Maimengdong tang)

Ingredients

Radix Ophiopogonis	30 g
Rhizoma Pinelliae	6 g
Radix Codonopsis Pilosulae	10 g
Radix Glycyrrhizae	3 g
Oryzae Sativae	10 g
Fructus Ziziphi Jujubae	4 pcs

Decoct the above ingredients in a right amount of water for oral administration.

Efficacy

Benefiting the stomach – qi and promoting the production of body fluid, lowering the adverse rising qi; mainly for cases of consumptive pulmonary diseases manifested by productive cough, shortness of breath, dry mouth and throat, red uncoated tongue, weak and rapid pulse, which are attributive to asthenia – heat of the stomach and adverse rising of qi and fire.

Indications

1. Indicated for cases of requent retching, accompanied with loss of appetite, dry mouth and throat, red and dry tongue, small and rapid pulse, which are attributive to insufficiency of stomach – yin and adverse rising of stomach – qi.

Also for cases of diabetes involving the middle – jiao, manifested by polyphagia, emaciation, red uncoated tongue, small, smooth and rapid pulse, which are atributive to insufficiency of stomach – yin and adverse rising of qi and fire.

Another prescription recorded in *Records of Traditional Chinese and Western Medicine in Combination* is composed of by omitting *Oryzae Sativae* and adding *Rhizoma Dioscoreae*, *Radix Paeoniae Alba*, *Cortex Moutan Radicis*, *Semen Persicae* to this prescription, applicable to retrograde menstruation.

4. Also applicable to cases of pulmonary tuberculosis, pleurisy, bronchiectasis, gastritis, gastric ulcer, hyperthyroidism, diabetes mellitus, etc. which are attributive to asthenic heat of stomach and adverse rising of qi and fire.

Interpretation

Ophiopogonis not only clears away asthenic heat from the lung and stomach, but also nourishes the yin – fluid of lung and stomach, and serves as the principal drug of the prescription. *Codonopsis Pilosulae*, *Glycyrrhizae*, *Ziziphi Jujubae* and *Oryzae Sativae* are applied to invigorate the qi and yin of spleen and stomach, and provide fluid for the lung.

Decoction of Perillae for Keeping Energy Downward
(Suzi jiangqi tang)

Ingredients

Fructus Perillae 10 g

Rhizoma Pinelliae Praeparata	10 g
Radix Peucedani	6 g
Cortex Magnoliae Officinalis	6 g

Decoct the above ingredients in a right amount of water for oral administration.

Efficacy

Lowering the abnormally rising of energy and relieving dyspnea, warming the kidney and promoting respiration; mainly for cases due to failure of kidney – qi to regulate inspiration (asthenia in the lower) or retention of cold – phlegm in the lung (sthenia in the upper), which are manifested by dyspneic cough, shortness of breath, wheezing, feeling of oppression over the chest, thin and clear sputum, whitish and smooth fur on the tongue.

Indications

1. This prescription is originally applied for dyspneic cough, which is sthenia in the upper and asthnia in the lower. Nowadays, it is also applicable to dyspneic cough of wind – cold type. When the cases are complicated by wind – cold superficial syndrome, add *Herba Ephedrae*, *Semen Armeniacae Amarum* to open the inhibited lung – qi and relieve dyspnea.

2. Also applicable to bronchial asthma, cardiac asthma, chronic bronchitis, emphysema, etc. marked by asthma or cough, which are attributive to sthenia in the upper and asthenia in the lower or retention of cold – phlegm in the lung.

Interpretation

Perillae is the chief drug in the prescription, and has the effects of lowering the abnormally rising energy, eliminating phlegm and relieving cough. *Pinelliae*, *Citri*, *Grandis*, *Magnoliae Officinalis* and *Peucedani* are helpful to ease the chest. *Angelicae*

Sinensis helps *Cinnamomi* to warm the kidney and promote respiration. *Glycyrrhizae* serves to regulate the above drugs.

Decoction of Phragmitis
(Weijing tang)

Ingredients

Rhizoma Phragmitis	60 g
Semen Coicis	30 g
Semen Benincasae	30 g
Semen Persicae	10 g

Decoct the above ingredients in a right amount of water for oral administration.

Efficacy

Clearing away lung – heat and eliminating sputum, removing blood stasis and pus; mainly for cases of pulmonary abscess with expectoration of foul, purulent and bloody sputum, chest pain aggravated by coughing, red tongue with yellow, greasy fur, smooth and rapid pulse.

Indications

1. This is a typical prescription for pulmonary abscess. For cases without formation of pus, add *Radix Platycodi* and *Bulbus Fritillariae Cirrhosae* to enhance the effect of eliminating the sputum and the pus.

2. For cases of measles after the occurrence of skin eruptions, but still with fever, productive cough, red tongue with yellow greasy fur, smooth and rapid pulse, which are attributive to lung – heat, omit *Persicae* and add *Cortex Mori Radicis* and *Bulbus Fritillariae Thunbergii*.

3. *Also applicable to cases of lobar pneumonia, bronchitis, whooping cough, etc. which are attributive to lung – heat.*

Interpretation

Phragmitis has the effects of clearing away lung – heat and is the principal remedy for pulmonary abscess. *Benincasae* eliminates sputum and pus. *Coicis* clears away heat – evil and promotes diuresis. *Persciae* removes blood stasis and pus. All of these three seeds can also move the bowels and eliminate the pus and blood stasis through defecation. These constitute and ideal prescription for pulmonary abscess of sputum – heat pattern or sputum – blood – stasis pattern. The abscess can be dispersed when the pus is not yet formed, and the pus can be eliminated when the abscess is formed.

Decoction of Pinellia and Magnolia Bark
(Banxia houpo tang)

Ingredients

Rhizoma Pinelliae	12 g
Cortex Magnoliae Officinalis	9 g
Poria	12 g
Rhizoma Zingiberis Recens	9 g
Folium Perillae	6 g

Decoct the above ingredients in a right amount of water for oral administration.

Efficacy

Promoting the circulation of qi to alleviate mental depression, lowering the adverse flow of qi and resolving phlegm.

Indications

Globus hystericus marked by a subjective sensation as if a plum pit is stuck in the throat which can neither be thrown up nor swallowed down, or accompanied by fullness and distress in the chest, and hypochondrium, or cough or vomiting, white, moist or greasy fur of the tongue, and slippery or taut pulse.

Pharyngoneurosis, neurogenic vomiting, gastric neurosis and vomiting of pregnancy marked by stagnancy of phlegm and qi or reversed flow of qi can be treated by the modified recipe.

The recip is mainly composed of drugs bitter and pungent in taste, warm and dry in nature, so it is only indicated for stagnation of phlegm and qi, partially for the phlegm – dampness. It is contraindicated in patients with deficiency of yin – fluid of hyperactivity of pathogenic fire due to yin deficiency.

Interpretation

Pinellia tuber in the recipe, with a pungent flavor and warm nature, is used as a principal drug to resolve phlegm, disperse stagnancy and regulate the stomach and lower the adverse flow of qi. *Magnolia bark*, pungent in flavor, bitter in tasted and warm in nature, can achieve the effects of sending down the ascending qi, relieving the sensation of fullness and assisting *Pinellia tuber* in dispersing stagnation and lowering the adverse flow of qi. *Poria*, sweet and bland in taste, can be used to induce diuresis and assist *Pinellia tuber* in resolving phlegm. The two drugs are regarded as assistant drugs. *Fresh ginger*, pungent in flavor and warm in nature, can be used to disperse stagnation, regulate the stomach and relieve vomiting. *Perilla leaf* promotes the circulation of qi, soothes the liver and regulates the spleen by means of its aroma. The two drugs are used as adjuvant drugs.

Modern researches have proved that the recipe has the effects of expelling phlegm, arresting cough, relieving spasm of smooth muscles of bronchus and regulating the function of autonomic nerve and removing edema.

Decoction of Poria, Cinnamomi, Atractyldis Macrocephalae and Glycyrrhizae (Fuling guizhi baizhu gancao tang)

Ingredients

Poria	20 g
Ramulus Cinnamomi	12 g
Rhizoma Atractylodis Macrocephalae	12 g
Radix Glycyrrhizae Praeparata	6 g

Decoct the above ingredients in a right amount of water for oral administration.

Efficacy

Strengthening spleen, promoting diuresis, warming yang – qi and eliminating phlegm; mainly for cases of phlegm – retention syndrome manifested by dizziness, fullness over the chest and hypochondrium, thirst without desire to drink, shortness of breath, cough, white and smooth or pale and greasy fur on the tongue, wiry and smooth pulse, etc., which are attributive to deficiency of middle – jiao yang and fluid retention.

Indications

1. This prescription is also effective for invigorating heart – yang. For cases of palpitation accompanied with fullness over the chest and epigastriu, cold limbs, fatigue, oliguria, thirst without desire to drink, whitish fur on the tongue, wiry pulse, which are attributive to declination of heart – yang and retention of fluid, the dosage of *Glycyrrhizae* may be increased to 10 g.

2. Applicable to cases of diarrhea with loose or watery stools, oliguria, white and smooth fur on the tongue, which are attributive to stagnation of cold – dampness in the spleen.

3. For cases of constipation accompanied with dry mouth but no desire to drink, corpulent and pale tongue with white and smooth fur, which are attributive to failure of the spleen to transport body fluid and dryness of intestines, *Atractylodis Macrocephalae* should be applied as crude rhizomes in large dosage (30 – 60 g).

4. Also applicable to cases of Meniere's syndrome, duodenal ulcer, cholecystitis, rheumatic heart diseases, chronic nephritis, etc., marked by dizziness, palpitation, and cases of bronchitis, emphysema, etc., marked by cough, which are attributive to deficiency of middle – jiao yang and retention of fluid, as well as cases of pulmonary tuberculosis, chronic gastritis, etc., marked by constipation, which are attributive to failure of the spleen to transport body fluid and dryness of intestines.

Interpretation

Poria can invigorate the spleen and eliminate dampness, and is used in a large dosage as the principal drug of the prescription. Since fluid retention is caused by the malfunction of vital qi which results from insufficiency of spleen – yang, so *Ramulus Cinnamomi* is applied for warming spleen – yang and promoting the circulation of vital qi. These two drugs used together have the effects of warming the spleen and eliminating dampness, and then relieving fluid retention. *Atractylodis Macrocephalae* can strengthen the spleen and benefit vital qi. It also can help *Poria* to eliminate dampness evil and inhibit the production of phlegm. *Glycyrrhizae Praeparata* can invigorate the spleen and benefit vital qi when it combines with *Atractylodis Macrocephalae* , and tonify yang when it combines with *Ramulus Cinnamomi*. Although the prescription has only four drugs, they match with each other reasonably, so that its effects is reliable and it is widely used clinically.

Decoction of Poria, Glycyrrhizae, Schisandrae, Zingiberis and Asari (Ling gan wuwei jiang xin tang)

Ingredients

Poria	15 g
Rhizoma Zingiberis	10 g
Herba Asari	6 g
Fructus Schisandrae	6 g
Radix Glycyrrhizae	6 g

Decoct the above ingredients in a right amount of water for oral administration.

Efficacy

Warming the lung and relieving phlegm – retention syndrome; mainly for cases attributive to insufficiency of spleen – yang and retention of phlegm in the interior, which are manifested by cough with whitish and thin sputu, salivation, feeling of oppression over the chest, vomiting, white and smooth fur on the tongue, sunken and slow pulse.

Indications

1. This prescription is suitable for syndrome attributive to retention of cold – phlegm in the lung. For cases with vomiting, retching or profuse expectoration, add *Pericarpium Citri Reticulatae* and *Fructus Amomi*; for cases with anorexia attributive to hypofunction of spleen, add *Atractylodis Macrocephalae* and *Rhizoma Dioscoreae*.

2. Applicable to cases of consumptive pulmonary diseases attributive to asthenia – cold of the lung and failure of fluid production by vital qi, which are manifested by cough with profuse expectoration of thin, clear sputum, dizziness, shortness of breath, fatigue, pale tongue, slow and weak pulse; in this case, *Zingiberis* and *Glycyrrhizae* serve to warm the lung and benefit vital qi.

3. Also applicable to cases of chronic bronchitis, emphysema, pulmonary tuberculosis, bronchiectasis, etc., which are attributive to retention of cold – phlegm in the lung.

Interpretation

Zingiberis has the effects of warming the lung and drying dampness to disperse phlegm, and serves as the main drug in the prescription. *Asari* has the effects of warming the lung to eliminate cold evil, and acts with *Zingiberis* to disperse the cold – phlegm. *Poria* can invigorate the spleen and eliminate dampness, and acts with *Zingiberis* to activate spleen – yang and inhibit the production of phlegm. *Fructus Schisandrae* exerts an astringent effect on the lung – qi and relieves cough, and also counteracts the lung – qi consuming effect of *Asari*. *Glycyrrhizae* can activate spleen – yang when it is accompanied by *Zingiberis*.

Decoction of Prepared Licorice (Zhigancao tang)

Ingredients

Radix Glycyrrhizae Praeparata	12 g
Rhizoma Zingiberis	9 g
Radix Ginseng	6 g
Radix Rehmanniae	30 g
Ramulus Cinnamomi	9 g
Colla Corii Asini	6 g
Radix Ophiopogonis	10 g
Fructus Cannabis	10 g
Fructus Ziziphi Jujubae	10 g

Decoct the above ingredients in a right amount of water for oral administration.

Efficacy

Replenishing qi, enriching the blood and nourishing yin to restore pulse.

Indications

Deficiency of both qi and blood manifested by regular intervals, or knotted pulse, or slow pulse with irregular intervals, palpitation, amaciation, shortness of breath, pallor, coat on the tongue with reduced saliva, frequent fever of deficiency type with unproductive cough, or with little expectoration of bloody sputum, insomnia due to vexation, spontaneous perspiration, or night sweat, dry mouth and throat, obstipation, and weak and rapid pulse.

Equally, other cases such as ventricular premature beat, primary stage of atrioventricular block, functional arrhythmia, auricular fibrillation, cardiovascular neurosis, hyperthyroidism, rheumatic heart disease and others that pertain to the deficiency of both qi and blood, can respond well to the modified recipe.

Interpretation

Acting as a principal drug in the recipe, the first ingredient gives the effect of enriching qi, replenishing the stomach and restoring the pulse. *Ginseng* together with *Ziziphi Jujubae*, is capable of nourishing the heart and spleen by way of replenishing qi. *Dried rehmania root*, *Donkey – hide gelatin*, *Ophiopogon root* and *Hemp seed*, all sweet in taste and moist in nature for nourishing yin and the heart, supplement the blood, moisten the lung and promote the production of body fluid. *Fresh ginger*, *Cinnamon twig* and *rice wine*, acrid in tasted and warm in property, are used for activating yang and restoring pulse, and in compatibility with drugs for replenishing qi and nourishing yin, they can gain the superiority of warmness without dryness, beneficial to promoting the flow of qi and the blood and easing the blood vessels.

Modern studies have ascertained that this recipe has the efficacies in increasing cerebral excitement, strengthening the function of heart, dilating the coronary artery.

Cautions

As the recipe has the effects of moistening dryness and relaxing the bowels, it is not suitable for patients with weakness of gastrointestine or with diarrhea.

Decoction of Rehmanniae and Lycii Radicis
(Liang di tang)

Ingredients

Radix Rehmanniae	30 g
Radix Scrophulariae	15 g
Radix Paeoniae Alba	15 g

Radix Ophiopogonis	9 g
Cortex Lycii Radicis	9 g
Colla Corii Asini	12 g

Decoct the above ingredients in a right amount of water for oral administration.

Efficacy

Nourishing kidney – yin and clearing away asthenic heat; mainly for cases with preceded menstrual cycle, discharge of small amount of thick and bright red menses, flushed cheeks, feverish sensation over the palms and soles, diziness, tinnitus, red tongue, small and rapid pulse, which are attributive to consumption of kidney – yin and stirring of asthenic fire inside the body.

Indications

1. Applicable to cases with metrorrhagia, discharge of bright red and thick bloody fluid from the vagina, flushed cheeks, restlessness, red tongue with a little of fur, small and rapid pulse, which are attributive to yin – deficiency and blood – heat.

2. Also indicated for consumptive diseases manifested by hectic fever, flushed cheeks, sore – throat, flaccidity of lower limbs, night sweat, crimson and uncoated tongue, sunken and small, weak pulse, which are attributive to insufficiency of kidney – yin and flamming up of asthenic fir.

3. Also applicable to tuberculosis of female reproductive organs, chronic hepatitis, Addisons disease, dysfunctional uterine bleeding, etc., attributive to consumption of kidney – yin or yin – deficiency and blood – heat.

Interpretation

Rehmanniae can nourish yin, promote the production of body fluid, clear away heat and cool the blood, and is used in large dosage and serves as the chief component of the prescription. *Scrophulariae* and *Ophiopogonis* also can nourish yin; *Paeoniae Alba* and *Colla Corii Asini* can nourish blood and promote the production of body fluid. The above four drugs serve to invigorate yin and keep yin and yang in equilibrium. *Lycii Radicis* clears away the asthenic heat of liver and kidney. In sum this prescription is designed for nourishing yin as the chief purpose, and clearing away heat as subsidiary, so that yin and yang are kept in equilibrium, the menstrual cycle will be restored to normal.

Decoction of Stephaniae Tetrandrae
(Mufangji tang)

Ingredients

Radix Stephaniae Tetrandrae	12 g
Ramulus Cinnamomi	10 g
Radix Codonopsis Pilosulae	10 g
Gypsum Fibrosum	30 g

Decoct the above ingredients in a right amount of water for oral administration.

Efficacy

Activating circulation of body fluid, dispersing stagnation, dredging the passage of yang – qi, lowering the adverse rising qi, and clearing away lung – heat; mainly for fluid – retention syndrome characterized by dyspnea and edema, accompanied by feeling of oppression over the chest, and hypochondrium, dull complexion, extreme thirst, yellow fur on the tongue, sunken and tense pulse, which are attributive to retention of fluid in the chest with weakness of healthy vital energy and hyperactivity of evil.

Indications

1. For bi – syndrome attributive to stagnation of dampness – heat in the meridians, which is manifested by erythema, swelling, pain and heat over the joints, fever, sweating, oliguria, yellow and greasy fur on the tongue, smooth and rapid pulse, omit *Codonopsis Pilosulae* and add *Semen Coicis* and *Rhizoma Atractylodis* to invigorate spleen and eliminate dampness.

2. Also applicable to cases of pleurisy, acute nephritis, emphysema complicated by infection, etc. marked by dyspnea, which are attributive to fluid retention in the thorax.

Interpretation

Stephaniae Tetrandrae eliminates the fluid retention, and *Ramulus Cinnamomi* warms the bladder. They act together to discharge the fluid retained in the thorax through diuresis. *Gypsum Fibrosum* can clear away lung – heat, and *Cinnamomi* can warm and activate the yang – qi of the thorax. The two help each other to release the stagnated lung

-qi, activate the fluid circulation and eliminate the heat evil. *Codonopsis Pilosulae* is applied to benefit and invigorate the lung and spleen, and also supplement vital qi with the help of *Cinnamomi*. It also prevent the damage of stomach by using *Gypsum Fibrosum*.

Decoction of Three Kinds of Seed for the Aged
(Sanzi yangqin tang)

Ingredients

Semen Sinapis Albae	6 g
Fructus Perillae	9 g
Semen Raphani	9 g

Decoct the above ingredients in a right amount of water for oral administration.

Efficacy

Sending down the abnormally ascending qi to relieve the discomfort in the chest, and resolving phlegm and promoting digestion.

Indications

Stagnation of phlegm and qi marked by cough, dyspnea, abundant expectoration and feeling of stuffiness in the chest, poor appetite and dyspepsia, whitish greasy tongue fur and slippery pulse.

Chronic bronchitis, bronchiectasis, bronchial asthma, pulmonary emphysema, cardiac asthma and other diseases marked by the syndrome of stagnation of phlegm and qi can be treated by the modified recipe.

Interpretation

White mustard seed in the recipe warms the lung and promotes the flow of qi, relieves chest discomfort and resolves phlegm. *Perilla fruit* lowers the adverse flow of qi and removes phlegm to arrest cough and relieve asthma. *Radish seed* promotes digestion to remove food stagnancy, and promotes the circulation of qi to eliminate phlegm.

Modern researches have proved that the recipe has the effects of eliminating phlegm, relieving cough and dyspnea, inducing diuresis, promoting gastrointestinal peristalsis and digestive and absorptive functions.

Cautions

When effective result is obtained after administration, the cause of the disease should be taken into consideration in the treatment.

Decoction of Trichosanthis and Allii Macrostemi
(Gualou xiebai baijiu tang)

Ingredients

Fructus Trichosanthis	15 g
Bulbus Allii Macrostemi	10 g
Rice wine	15 g

Decoct the above ingredients in a right amount of water for oral administration.

Efficacy

Easing the chest, eliminating phlegm, activating yang – qi and dispersing stagnation; mainly for cases of chest bi – syndrome due to stagnation of phlegm and declination of yang – qi in the chest, which are manifested by dull aching over the chest which may be referred to the back, whitish and greasy fur on the tongue, sunken and wiry pulse.

Indications

1. For cases with productive cough, chest pain referring to the back, whitish and greasy fur on the tongue, which are attributed to the stagnation of phlegm and declination of chest – yang, omit the rice wine and add *Radix Asteris* and *Flos Farfarae* to eliminate phlegm and relieve cough.

2. For cases with chest pain referring to the back and aggravated by cold, sunken and slow pulse, which are attributed to a serious attack of cold evil, add *Rhizoma Zingiberis* and *Herba Asari* to warm the lung and eliminate the cold evil.

3. Generally the dosage of rice wine is 15 – 60 ml, and should be decreased when the patient cannot tolerate.

4. Also applicable to cases of angina pectoris, intercostal neuralgia, chronic bronchi-

tis, etc. which are attributive to stagnation of phlegm and declination of chest – yang.

Interpretation

Trichosanthis, bitter in flavour and cold in nature, has the effects of eliminating phlegm and easing the chest. *Allii Macrostemi*, acrid in flavour and warm in nature, has the effect of activating yang – qi of the chest. When used together, they are superior to eliminate phlegm, dampness and other yin – evils. *Rice wine* has the effects of promoting the blood and vital qi circulation and enhancing the yang – activating effect of *Allii Macrostemi*. As a whole, the prescription aims at eliminating phlegm and activating yang, thus the vital qi function normally and the chest pain will be relieved.

Decoction with Direct Effect on Moyuan
(Da yuan yin)

Ingredients

Semen Arecae	12 g
Cortex Magnoliae Officinalis	9 g
Rhizoma Anemarrheane	9 g
Radix Paeoniae Alba	9 g
Radix Scutellariae	9 g
Fructus Tsaoko	6 g
Radix Glycyrrhizae	6 g

Decoct the above ingredients in a right amount of water for oral administration.

Efficacy

Expelling pathogenic factor at moyuan, eliminating dampness evil; mainly for pestilence or malaria attributive to retention of dampness – heat evil in moyuan, manifested by chilliness and high fever once or three times daily, vomiting, nausea, headache, irritability, dark – red tongue with turbid and greasy fur, wiry and rapid pulse.

Indications

1. For cases of syncope resulting from crapulence, manifested by abdominal flatu-

lence, sudden fainting, cold limbs, sweating over the forehead, thick and yellowish, greasy fur on the tongue, smooth and solid pulse, add *Rhizoma Acori Graminei* and omit *Glycyrrhizae* from this prescription.

2. For cases of diarrhea with discharge of foul stools, abdominal pain and fullness, yellowish and greasy fur on the tongue, smooth and rapid pulse, which are attributive to stagnation of dampness - heat evil in the middle - jiao, add *Rhizoma Coptidis*, *Talcum* and omit *Glycyrrhizae*, *Paeoniae Alba*.

3. Also applicable to cases of influenza, malaria, septicemia attributive to retention of dampness - heat evil in moyuan, also to cases of vegetative neurosis, indigestion, acute enteritis attributive to retention of dampness and heat evil.

Interpretation

Tsaoko has the effects of eliminating dampness, stopping vomiting and letting out the hidden evil. *Magnoliae Officinalis* serves to disperse dampness, promote circulation ov vital qi and dredge the stagnation. *Arecae* dissipates phlegm - dampness, activates vital qi and relieve the accumulation of heat evil. All the three drugs serve as the chief drugs acting directly on moyuan to let out the evils. *Scutellariae* and *Anemarrhenae* purge the fire and eliminate toxic material. *Paeoniae Alba* and *Glycyrrhizae* serve as to enhance the action of *Scutellariae* and *Anemarrhenae* and prevent the damage of yin - essence.

Ephedrae Decoction
(Mahuang tang)

Ingredients

Herba Ephedrae	6 g
Ramulus Cinnamomi	4 g
Semen Armeniacae Amarum	9 g
Radix Glycyrrhizae Praeparata	3 g

Decoct the above ingredients in a right amount of water for oral administration.

Efficacy

Inducing sweat to relieve exterior syndrome, facilitating the flow of the lung - qi to relieve asthma.

Indications

Exterior syndrome of excess type due to exopathic wind - cold marked by aversion to cold, fever without perspiration, headache, pantalgia, dyspnea, thin and white coating of the tongue, superficial and tight pulse.

Moreover, the recipe can be modified to deal with cold, influenza, bronchitis, bronchial asthma and others that are ascribed to exterior syndrome of excess type caused by exopathic wind - cold.

Interpretation

In the recipe, *Ephedra*, pungent and bitter in flavour and slight warm in nature, acts as a principal drug with the effect of inducing sweat to dispel exogenous evils and facilitating the flow of the lung - qi to relieve asthma. *Cinnamon twig*, pungent and sweet in flavour and warm in nature, has the effects of warming and dredging the blood vessels and activating the heart - yang and serves as an assistant drug that helps strengthen the effect of the principal drug. Possessing bitter and pungent flavour and warm nature, *Bitter apricot kernel* is used as an adjuvant drug with the effect of arresting cough and relieving asthma. *Prepared licorice root* is an ingredient sweet in flavour and warm in nature and functions as a guiding drug, having the effects of reinforcing the middle - warmer, replenishing qi, moistening the lung to relieve cough and tempering the effect of other drugs.

Clinically and experimentally, it is ascertained that this recipe can relieve the troubles by producing the effects of inducing sweat, removing fever, arresting cough, relieving pain and promoting diuresis.

Cautions

1. Being warm and pungent, the recipe is drastic in its effect of inducing sweat, so it should not be administered for cases that have nothing to do with exterior syndrome of excess type due to expathic wind - cold such as spontaneous perspiration caused by exterior syndrome of deficiency type, general debility with exogenous diseases, blood deficiency after giving birth, etc..

2. As soon as sweat is induced out and the illness is cured, the administration should be withdrawn immediately. Prolongation of intake is of no benefit.

Jade Screen Powder

Ingredients

Radix Astragali seu Hedysari	30 g
Rhizoma Atractylodis Macrocephalae	10 g
Radix Ledebouriellae	10 g

Decoct the above ingredients in a right amount of water for oral administration.

Efficacy

Benefiting vital qi, eliminating pathogenic agents, strengthening the superficial resistance and stopping sweating; mainly for those who are liable to be affected by wind and cold due to deficiency of vital qi and weakness of superficial resistance, and for cases of spontaneous sweating with pale complexion, pale tongue with whitish fur, floating and weak pulse.

Indications

1. For debilitated persons who are suffering from mild comon cold of wind – cold type, manifested by aversion to wind, sweating, pale tongue with whitish fur, floating and weak pulse, add *Ramulus Cinnamomi* to expel the cold evil from the muscles.

2. For cases of urticaria with pale tongue, whitish fur, floating and weak pulse, which are attributive to deficiency of vital qi and attack of wind evil, add *Radix Angelicae Sinensis* to activate blood circulation to expel the wind evil.

3. Also applicable to cases of common cold, neurodermatitis, urticaria, allergic rhinitis, etc., which are attributive to deficiency of vital qi with affection of wind. Also used for the prevention of common cold.

Interpretation

Astragali seu Hedysari can greatly tonify primordial qi of the spleen and lung. When primordial qi is full, the superficial resistance will be strengthened and sweating arrested. so it is used in larger dosage and serves as the principal drugs. The lung controls vital qi which originates from foods, so that *Macrocephalae* is used for tonifying the spleen to promote the production of vital qi and blood. Although spontaneous sweating results from the weakness of superficial resistance, but it is connected with the attack of wind evil, *Ledebouriellae is used for eliminating wind evil. In the prescription*, *Astragali seu hedysari* is helped by *Ledebouriellae* to get rid of the exogenous wind, and *Macrocephalae* to invigorate the spleen and thus to strengthen the interior. It serves as a causative treatment for spontaneous sweating due to deficiency of vital qi. As to those who liable to catch cold, the primary cause is the weakness of the uperficial resistance and not the wind evil. If the wind eliminating remedy is used only, the healthy qi will be damaged. The three ingredients used together can both support the healthy qi and eliminate the evils, so that common cold may be prevented.

Kuoqing Decoction
(Kuoqing yin)

Ingredients

Pericarpium Arecae	12 g
Poria	15 g
Fructus Aurantii	10 g
Cortex Magnoliae Officinalis	10 g
Semen Raphani	10 g
Rhizoma Alismatis	10 g
Semen Sinapis Alba	6 g
Pericarpium Citri Reticulatae	6 g

Decoct the above ingredients in a right amount of water for oral administration.

Efficacy

Eliminating dampness, promoting diuresis and activating vital qi; mainly for cases attributive to retention of phlegm – dampness in the triple jiao, manifested by fullness over the chest, shortness of breath, dyspnea, general edema, oliguria, white and greasy fur on the tongue, smooth pulse.

Indications

1. Applicable to cases with abdominal distension, poor appetite, eructation, oliguria, white and greasy fur on the tongue, wiry pulse, which are attributive to the stagnation of

vital qi and dampness.

2. Also indicated for cases of sinusitis with turbid and thick nasal discharge, white and greasy fur on the tongue, wiry pulse, which are attributive to the affection of phlegm – dampness to the nasal orifice.

3. Also applicable to cases of chronic cor pulmonale and chronic nephritis with dyspnea, cough and edema attributive to stagnation of phlegm – dampness in the triple jiao; and to cases of cirrhotic of ascites attributive to the stagnation of vital qi and dampness.

Interpretation

Poria and *Alismatis* can eliminate dampness by promoting diuresis. *Arecae* serves to enhance the diuretic effect of the above drugs by activating vital qi. *Aurantii*, *Citri Reticulatae* and *Magnoliae Officinalis* can promote the circulation of vital qi. *Sinapis Alba* and *Raphani* serve to regulate the vital qi and eliminate the sputum retained in the upper jiao, and also soothe the chest and relieve the stagnation of vital qi when combined with the above drugs.

Lophatherum and Gypsum Decoction
(Zhuye shigao tang)

Ingredients

Herba Lophatheri	15 g
Gypsum Fibrosum	30 g
Rhizoma Pinelliae Praeparata	9 g
Radix ophiopogonis	15 g
Radix Ginseng	5 g
Radix Glycyrrhizae Praeparata	3 g
Semen Oryzae Nonglutinosae	15 g

Decoct the above ingredients in a right amount of water for oral administration.

Efficacy

Clearing away heat and promoting the production of body fluid, replenishing qi and regulating the stomach.

Indications

Lingering heat with impairment of both the qi and body fluid in the later stage of exogenous febrile disease, epidemic febrile disease and summer – heat disease, marked by feverish body, hyperhidrosis, general debility and short breath, irritability, inclination to vomit, dry mouth and fondness of drink, or insomnia due to restlessness, reddened tongue with little coating, and rapid pulse.

The recipe can also be modified to deal with cases with deficiency of both qi and yin occuring in the later stage of influenza, epidemic encephalitis B epidemic cerebrospinal meningitis, pneumonia and septicemia.

Interpretation

In the recipe, *Lophatherum* and *Gypsum*, with the effects of clearing away heat and relieving restlessness, are used as principal drugs. *Ophiopogon root* and *Ginseng*, being effective for nourishing yin and promoting the production of body fluid, serve as assistant drugs. *Prepared pinelia tuber* is an adjuvant drug for lowering the adverse flow of qi to relieve vomiting. *Prepared licorice root* and *Polished round – grained nonglutinous rice* are guiding drugs with the functions nourishing the stomach and regulating the middle – warmer.

Clinically and experimentally, it is ascertained that the recipe is contributive not only to nourishing and strengthening the constitution to promote digestion and absorption, but also to subduing inflammation, tranquilizing the mind, bringing down fever, arresting cough, dispelling phlegm and preventing vomiting.

Cautions

It is not advisable for cases with febrile disease when the vital qi is dominating with pathogens prevailing, or excessive heat existing in the body, or neither qi nor yin being impaired.

Minor Decoction of Bupleurum
(Xiao chaihu tang)

Ingredients

Radix Bupleuri	12 g
Radix Scutellariae	9 g
Rhizoma Pinelliae	9 g
Rhizoma Zingiberis Recens	9 g
Radix Ginseng	6 g
Fructus Ziziphi Jujubae	4 pcs
Radix Glycyrrhizae Praeparata	5 g

Decoct the above ingredients in a right amount of water for oral administration.

Efficacy

Treating *shaoyang* disease by mediation.

Indications

Shaoyang disease with the pathogenic factors located neither in the exterior nor in the interior but in between marked by alternate attacks of chills and fever, fullness in the chest, hypochondriac discomfort, anorexia, dysphoria, retching, bitterness in the mouth, dry throat, dizziness, thin and white fur on the tongue and stringy pulse, or exogenous febrile diseases occcuring in women belonging to invasion of the blood chamber by pathogenic heat.

The common cold, malaria, infection of biliary tract, hepatitis, pleuritis, chronic gastritis, indigestion, mastosis, intercostal neuralgia, neurosis and AIDS marked by the symptoms of *shaoyang* disease can be treated by the modified recipe.

Interpretation

Bupleurum root, as a principal drug, dispels the pathogenic factor located in the half exterior by driving it out. *Scutellaria root* clears out stagnated heat located in the half interior by clearing away it thoroughly as an assistant drug. The combined use of the two drugs, one for dispelling pathogen, and the other for clearing away stagnated heat, removes pathogenic factors from *shaoyang* channels. *Pinellia tuber* and *Fresh ginger* regulate the function of the stomach and lower the adverse flow of qi. *Ginseng* and *Chinese dates* invigorate qi and strengthen the middle – warmer. *Prepared licorice root* coordinates the actions of various drugs in the recipe. *Pinellia tuber* and *Prepared licorice root* act as adjuvant and guiding drugs.

Modern researches have proved that the recipe has some effects of inhibiting bacteria, viruses and leptospira, relieving the reaction of the human body to the invaded pathogen, and remarkably allaying fever and resisting inflammation. In addition, the recipe also has the effects of promoting digestion, preventing vomiting, expelling phlegm, relieving cough, protecting the liver, normalizing the functioning of the gallbladder and tranquilizing the mind.

Cautions

Patients with syndromes such as upper excess with lower deficiency, or excess of liver – fire, hyperactivity of the liver – yang, hematemesis due to deficiency of yin are forbidden to use the recipe.

Minor White Powder of Three Drugs (Sanwu xiaobai san)

Ingredients

Fructus Crotonis
Radix Platycodi
Bulbus Fritillariae Cirrhosae

Efficacy

Inducing vomiting of sthenic phlegm and purging the accumulated cold; mainly for cases attributive to accumulation of cold in the ches and retention of phlegm – dampness in the lung, which manifest distending pain and tenderness of the chest and hypochondrium, profuse expectoration, dyspnea or cough with thick purulent sputum, constipation, white and greasy fur on the tongue, sunken and slow or sunken and tense pulse.

Indications

1. Applicable to cases with retention of sputum in the throat, dyspnea, dysphonia, or even trismus and unconsciousness, turbid and greasy fur on the tongue, sunken and tense pulse, which are attributive to accumulation of phlegm in the lung and dysfunction of vital qi.

2. Also applicable to cases of bronchiectasis complicated by infection and lung abscess, which are attributive to accumulation of cold in the thorax; and to cases of laryngeal diphtheria, peritonsillar abscess and retropharyngeal abscess, which are attributive to accumulation of phlegm in the lung and dysfunction of vital qi.

Interpretation

Platycodi not only can release the inhibited lung-qi but also can expel phlegm and pus. *Bulbus Fritillariae Cirrhosae* is applied for eliminating phlegm-dampness from the chest. *Crotonis* can expel cold by purgation. *Platycodi* has an ascending effect while *Crotonis* has a descending effect. They two acting together can induce vomiting of phlegm-dampness and also purge the accumulated cold. This prescription and the *Pill of Three Drugs for Emergency* both contain *Crotonis*, but the former is used for eliminating the cold retained in the chest while the latter for purging the cold accumulated in the intestines.

Modified Decoction of Fragrant Solmonseal Rhizome (Jiajian weirui tang)

Ingredients

Rhizoma Polygonati Odorati	9 g
Bulbus Allii Fistulosi	6 g
Radix Platycodi	5 g
Radix Cynanchi Atrati	3 g
Semen Sojae Praeparatum	9 g
Herba Menthae	5 g
Radix Glycyrrhizae Praeparata	2 g
Fructus Ziziphi Jujubae	2 pcs

Decoct the above ingredients in a right amount of water for oral administration.

Efficacy

Nourishing yin and clearing away heat, inducing sweat to relieve exterior syndrome.

Indications

Original yin – deficiency with re – affection due to exopathogen, manifested by headache, fever, light aversion to wind – cold, dry throat with cough, sputum too viscous to be coughed out, absence of sweat or little sweat, thirst and restlessness, reddened tongue and rapid pulse.

Moreover, the recipe can be modified to deal with the common cold, influenza, bronchitis and others that indicate exopathic diseases due to yin deficiency with re – affection by exopathogens after giving birth or bleeding.

Interpretation

Acting as a principal drug in the recipe, *Fragrant solomonseal rhizome* sweet in flavor and mildly moist in property, provides the effect of nourishing yin, promoting the production of body fluid in order to enrich the source of perspiration, moistening the lung to relieve cough, and eliminating pathogenic heat from the throat so as to allay pain. *Chinese green onion*, *Platycodon root*, *Prepared soybean* and *peppermint* together play the role of assistant drugs for relieving the exterior syndrome and facilitating the flow of lung – qi to relieve cough and sore throat. *Swallowwort root* and *Chinese date* are used in combination as adjuvant drugs; the former, having a bitter and salty taste and cold property, is used to quench thirst and get rid of irritability by cooling the blood and removing heat, and the latter, with a sweet flavour, exterts the effect of moistening and nourishing the spleen. *Prepared licorice root* is administered as a guiding drug for coordinating the effect of various drugs in the recipe.

Modern studies have confirmed that this recipe is qualified as tonics for consolidating the constitution and a curative one for inducing sweat, bringing down fever, subduing inflammation, relieving cough, expelling phlegm, etc..

Cautions

This recipe is only advisable for exogenous diseases with yin deficiency; it is contraindicated in cases without yin deficiency.

Notopterygium Decoction of Nine Ingredients (Jiuwei qianghuo tang)

Ingredients

Rhizoma Seu Radix Notopterygii	6 g
Radix Ledebouriellae	6 g
Rhizoma Atractylodis	6 g
Herba Asari	2 g
Rhizoma Ligustici Chuanxiong	3 g
Radix Angelicae Dahuricae	3 g
Radix Rehmanniae	3 g
Radix Scutellariae	3 g
Radix Glycyrrhizae	3 g

Decoct the above ingredients in a right amount of water for oral administration.

Efficacy

Relieving exterior syndrome, clearing interior heat and alleviating pain.

Indications

Syndrome due to the attack of exogenous wind, cold and dampness on the body surface with interior heat, manifested by chill and fever, absence of perspiration, headache with stiff neck, aching pain of the extremities, bitter taste in the mouth with thirst, white and slippery coating of the tongue, floating pulse, etc..

The recipe can be modified to deal with influenza, lumbago, sciatica rheumatic arthritis that are ascribable to the attack of exogenous wind-cold-dampness on the body surface with interior heat.

Interpretation

Of all the ingredients in the recipe, ***Notopterygium root***, possessing pungent, bitter and warm properties, acts as a principal drug for inducing diaphoresis, expelling pathogenic wind and dampness, removing stagnation of blood and qi and arresting pain; ***Ledebouriella*** and ***Atractylodes rhizome***, with the effects of inducing sweat and dispelling dampness, act as asistant drugs to reinforce the effect of ***Notopterygium root*** in dispelling exogenous evils; ***Asarum herb***, ***Chuanxiong rhizome*** and ***Dahurian angelica root*** are used together to dispel pathogenic cold and wind, promoting the flow of qi and blood and treating headache and pantalgia. As *Scutellaria root* exerts the effect of purging heat from the blood system, both of them are used as adjuvant drugs not only for the treatment of interior heat but also for the control of dryness due to pungent and warm properties of the drugs. *Licorice root* is used as a mediator for tempering the effect of other drugs in the recipe, playing the role of a guiding drug.

Modern researches have confirmed that the recipe has the efficacies in inducing diaphoresis, reducing fever, tr4anquilizing the mind, alleviating pain, promoting diuresis, and relieving inflammation.

Cautions

Patients with weakness of the vital qi and deficiency of yin are prohibited from taking the recipe.

Pill for Asthma
(Lengxiao wan)

Ingredients

Herba Ephedrae	10 g
Pericarpium Zanthoxyli	10 g
Rhizoma Pinelliae	10 g
Rhizoma Arisaema cum Bile	10 g
Semen Aremnicae Amarum	10 g
Herba Asari	3 g
Radix Glycyrrhizae	3 g
Radix Aconiti Praeparata	3 g
Alumen	2 g
Fructus Gleditsiae	2 g
Radix Asteris	15 g
Flos Farfarae	15 g
Rhizoma Zingiberis Recens	6 g
Massa Fermentata Medicinalis	6 g

Decoct the above ingredients in a right amount of water for oral administration.

Efficacy

Warming the lung, expelling cold and eliminating sputum; mainly for cases of cold–induced bronchial asthma with thin and whitish expectoration, feeling of oppression over the chest, white and smooth fur on the tongue, tense pulse, which are attributive to retention of cold–phlegm in the lung and impairment of its functional acitivities.

Indications

1. For cases of multiple abscesses with white and smooth fur on the tongue, sunken and slow pulse, which are attributive to the attack of dampness–phlegm, use *Semen Sinapis Albae* and *Cortex Cinnamomi* instead of *Asteris* and *Farfarae*.

2. Also applicable to cases of asthmatic bronchitis attributive to obstruction of the air passage by cold–phlegm, and those of cold abscess attributive to the attack of dampness–phlegm.

Interpretation

Ephedrae, *Aconiti Praeparata* and *Asari* have the effects of warming the lung and expelling cold. *Zanthoxyli* can warm the middle–jiao and eliminate dampness, they serve to deal with the cause of sputum production. *Alumen* and *Gleditsiae* are expectorants; *Pinelliae* and *Arisaema cum Bile* increase expectoration and ease the breathing; *Armeniacae Amarum*, *Asteris* and *Farfarae* are antitussives and antiasthmatics. This group of drugs serve to relieve the obstruction of air passage by the sputum. *Zingiberis Recens* can eliminate cold–phlegm and help *Gleditsiae* to expel sputum, and also counteracts the toxicity of *Aconiti Praeparata*. *Massa Fermentata Officinalis* is used for activating the spleen, promoting digestion and enhancing the expectorant effect of *Pinelliae*. *Glycyrrhizae* coordinates the action of other drugs and inhibits the poisonous effect of *Gleditsiae*.

Pill for Clearing Away Heat in Qifen and Dispersing Phlegm (Qingqi huatan wan)

Ingredients

Arisaema cum bile	12 g
Semen Trichosanthis	12 g

Rhizoma Pinelliae	10 g
Exocarpium Citri Grandis	10 g
Radix Scutellariae	10 g
Semen Armeniacae Amarum	10 g
Fructus Aurantii Immaturus	10 g
Poria	10 g
Rhizoma Zingiberis Recens	3 pcs

Decoct the above ingredients in a right amount of water for oral administration.

Efficacy

Clearing away heat evil, dispersing phlegm, lowering the adverse rising qi and relieving cough; mainly for cases attributive to stagnation of phlegm and heat in the lung, which are manifested by cough with difficult expectoration of thick yellow sputum, fullness over the chest, red tongue with yellow and greasy fur, smooth and rapid pulse, etc..

Indications

1. This prescription is a common recipe for the treatment of heat – phlegm. For cases with overabundance of lung – heat which may be manifested by yellow and dry fur on the tongue, omit *Pinelliae* and add *Gypsum Fibrosum* to purge the lung – heat. For cases with constipation attributive to the accumulation of heat evil, add *Rhizoma Polygoni Cuspidati* to purge heat evil, promote bowel movement and relieve cough.

2. Applicable to cases of nasosinusitis attributive to the stagnation of phlegm and heat which are manifested by prolonged discharge of yellow and foul fluid from the nose, yellow and greasy fur on the tongue, wiry and smooth pulse.

3. Also applicable to cases of bronchitis, pneumonia, emphysema, etc., marked by cough with yellow sputum, or cases of chronic rhinitis, which are attributive to the stagnation of phlegm and heat.

Interpretation

Arisaema cum Bile has the effects of eliminating phlegm and clearing away heat evil, and is used in large dosage and serves as the principal drug. *Trichosanthis* and *Scutellariae* enhance the expectorant effect of *Arisaema cum Bile*. *Aurantii Immaturus* and *Citri Grandis* are applied to lower the adverse qi and eliminate phlegm, and help

Trichosanthis to relieve cough. *Pinelliae* used together with *Arisaema cum Bile* and *Zingiberis Recens* is useful for eliminating the sputum which is produced already; while *Poria* used together with *Citri Grandis* can promote the function of spleen to eliminate dampness and then inhibit the production of sputum. *Armeniacae Amarum* has the effects of opening and lowering the lung – qi and relieving cough. When used together with *Trichosanthis*, it can promote bowel movement which is helpful for relieving cough and also counteract the dry nature of *Citri Grandis* and *Pinelliae* which may consume the body fluid.

Pill for Eliminating Phlegm Evil
(Gun tan wan)

Ingredients

Radix et Rhizoma Rhei (steamed with wine)	240 g
Radix Scutellariae (washed with wine)	240 g
Lignum Aquilariae Resinatum	15 g
Lapis Chloriti (roasted with Niter)	30 g

All ground into powder and prepared as pills.

Efficacy

Purging fire and eliminating phlegm; mainly for cases of chronic phlegm – syndrome of sthenic heat type, manifested by mania with frightening, or dyspneic cough with thick sputum, or feeling of oppression over the chest and epigastrium, or dizziness with profuse expectoration, constipation, yellow and thick, greasy fur on the tongue, smooth and rapid strong pulse.

Indications

1. This formula cannot be takeen as decoction.

2. Applicable to cases of nasosinusitis manifested by stuffy nose, headache, turbid, foul, thick and yellow nasal discharge, yellow and greasy fur on the tongue, wiry and rapid pulse, which are attributive to the attack of phlegm – heat from the spleen and stomach to the nasal orifice.

3. Applicable to cases of chronic suppurative otitis media accompanied with deafness, tinnitus, yellow and greasy fur on the tongue, wiry and rapid pulse, which are attributive to the attack of dampness – heat (or phlegm – heat0 of liver and gallbladder to the orifice.

4. Also applicable to cases of schizophrenia, manic – depressive psychosis, chronic bronchitis, emphysema, etc., which are attributive to chronic phlegm – syndrome of sthenic heat type.

Interpretation

Lapis Chloriti is a potent drug for lowering vital qi and phlegm. *Niter*, which roasted with *Lapis Chloritis* serve to enhance the phlegm – eliminating effect of the latter. *Lignum Aquilariae Resinatum* can lower the abnormal energy, and guide the phlegm – fire downward. *Rhei* and *Scutellariae* used together serve to purge phlegm – fire from the feces. In this prescription, there are drugs of bitter – cold (*Rhei* and *Scutellariae*), bitter – warm (*Aquilariae Resinatum*) and salty – bland (*Lapis Chloriti*), they counteract but an effect of lowering fire and eliminating phlegm is obtained.

Pill of Dioscoreae
(Shuyu wan)

Ingredients

Rhizoma Dioscoreae	15 g
Radix Rehmanniae	15 g
Radix Angelicae Sinensis	6 g
Ramulus Cinnamomi	6 g
Rhizoma Ligustici Chuanxiong	6 g
Radix Ophiopogonis	6 g
Radix Paeoniae Alba	6 g
Rhizoma Atractylodis Macrocephalae	6 g
Semen Sojae Germinatus	10 g
Radix Codonopsis Pilosulae	10 g
Poria	10 g
Colla Corii Asini (dissolved)	10 g
Massa Fermentata Officinalis	3 g
Radix Glycyrrhizae	3 g

Semen Armeniacae Amarum	3 g
Radix Bupleuri	3 g
Radix Platycodi	3 g
Rhizoma Zingiberis	3 g
Radix Ampelopsis	3 g
Radix Ledebouriellae	3 g
Fructus Ziziphi Jujubae	6 pcs

Decoct the above ingredients in a right amount of water for oral administration.

Efficacy

Expelling wind and tonifying; mainly for consumptive diseases complicated by the attack of wind evil, manifested by dizziness, emaciation, fatigue, shortness of breath, spontaneous sweat, alternate feeling of chills and fever, liability to cathc cold, poor appetite, loose stools, sallow complexion, aple tongue with white fur, soft and weak pulse, which are attributive to deficiency of lung – and spleen – qi, decrease of body resistance and impairment of healthy qi.

Indications

1. Applicable to cases with migratory arthralgia, emaciation, fatigue, sallow complexion, pale tongue with white and greasy smooth fur, feeble pulse, which are attributive to attack of wind – cold – dampness to the meridians and the impairment of healthy vital qi.

2. Also applicable to cases of pulmonary tuberculosis and emphysema, attributive to consumption of healthy vital qi and attack of wind; and to cases of rheumatic arthritis and gouty arthritis attributive to attack of the meridians by wind – cold – dampness and the impairment of healthy vital qi.

Interpretation

Dioscoreae acts as the principal drug in the prescription, which has the effects of invigorating spleen and benefiting the lung. *Codonopsis Pilosulae*, *Atractylodis Macrocephalae*, *Poria*, *Glycyrhizae*, *Zingiberis* and *Ziziphi Jujubae* are applied for strengthening the spleen and benefiting vital qi. *Ligustici Chuanxiong*, *Angelicae Sinensis*, *Paeoniae Alba*, *Rehmanniae*, *Ophiopogonis* and *Colla Corii Asini* can nourish the yin－blood. They all together serve to increase the tonic effect of *Dioscoreae*. *Massa Fermentat Officinalis* and *Sojae Germinatus* are used for promoting the function of spleen and eliminating dampness; *Armeniacae Amarum* and *Platycodi* for soothing the lung－qi. *Ledebouriellae*, *Ramulus Cinnamomi*, *Bupleuri* and *Ampelopsis* are selected to expel wind, and then to restore the healthy vital qi.

Pill of Six Miraculous Drugs
(Liushen wan)

Ingredients

Margarita	4.5 g
Calculus Bovis	4.5 g
Moschus	4.5 g
Realgar	3 g
Borneolum Syntheticum	3 g
Venenum Bufonis	3 g

Coated with burnt herbal powder.

Efficacy

Clearing away heat and toxic material, relieving swelling and alleviating pain; mainly for cases of scarlet fever and tonsillitis with red tongue and rapid pulse, which are attributive to the accumulation of phlegm, fire and toxic material.

Indications

1. The prescription cannot be applied as a decoction for oral use. Some ingredients such as *Realgar* and *Venenum Bufonis* are poisonous, so it should not be taken in alrge dose nor for a long period and is contraindicated for pregnant women.

2. Applicable to carbuncle, furuncle, abscess of breast, and various local infection of unknown origin, which are attributive to accumulation of phlegm, fire and toxic material.

3. Also applicable to cases of pharyngitis, follicular stomatitis, mastitis, nasopharyngeal carcinoma, lung cancer, etc. which are attributive to accumulation of phlegm, fire and toxic material.

Interpretation

Calculus Bovis, *Realgar* and *Venenum Bufonis* are principal drugs in the prescription, which have strong and fast effect of eliminating toxic materials and dispersing the accumulation of evils. *Calculus Bovis* can eliminate heat – phlegm, *Realgar* can disperse the stagnated substance, and *Venenum Bufonis* can relieve swelling and alleviate pain. They all are potent agents for clearing away heat and dispelling toxic material, and serve as the principal drugs of the prescription. *Margarita* can clear away heart – fire and eliminate phlegm when it combines with *Calculus Bovis*. *Borneolum Syntheticum* can disperse heat and alleviate pain, and also increase the effect of the other drugs with it combining with *Moschus*. *Burnt herbal powder* has the effect of dispersing the stagnated substance and easing the throat, and is especially good for the infection of oral cavity. In sum, the prescription has a strong detoxifying and swelling – subsiding effect by utilizing the fragrant nature of the ingredients.

Powder Containing Nine Drugs
(Jiuxian san)

Ingredients

Radix Codonopsis Pilosulae	12 g
Colla Corii Asini	12 g
Flos Farfarae	12 g
Cortex Mori Radicis	12 g
Pericarpium Papaveris (prepared with honey)	10 g
Fructus Mume	10 g
Bulbus Fritillariae Cirrhosae	10 g
Fructus Schisandrae	6 g
Radix Platycodi	6 g

Decoct the above ingredients in a right amount of water for oral administration.

Efficacy

Benefiting vital qi, invigorating the lung, keeping lung – qi and relieving cough; mainly for cases attributive to deficiency of lung – qi and failure of keeping lung – qi, which are manifested by chronic cough, shortness of breath, spontaneous sweating, tender and red tongue, feeble and rapid pulse.

Indications

1. This is a common recipe applied for prolonged cough, dyspnea and spontaneous sweating attributive to the consumption of yin and vital qi. For cases accompanied with hectic fever, add *Cortex Lycii Radicis* to clear away asthenic heat.

2. For cases of chronic diarrhea or dysentery with fecal incontinence, fatigue, tender and red tongue, small and rapid weak pulse, omit *Fritillariae Cirrhosae* and *Farfarae* from this prescription.

3. Also applicable to cases of pulmonary tuberculosis, emphysema, laryngophthisis, whooping cough, bronchiectasis, silicosis, etc. marked by prolonged cough, which are attributive to deficiency of lung - qi.

Interpretation

Papaveris is effective for keeping lung - qi and relieving cough. *Mume* and *Schisandrae* enhance the effect of *Papaveris* and also prevent the consumption of lung - qi; three drugs constituent a strong antitussive remedy. *Platycodi* lifts up the lung - qi. *Farfarae*, *Mori Radicis* and *Fritillariae Cirrhosae* serve to eliminate phlegm and relieve cough. *Codonopsis Pilosulae* is applied to invigorate lung - qi which may be impaired after prolonged cough. *Colla Corii Asini* is used for nourishing lung - yin. In sum this prescription serve to keep lung - qi in pure and descendant, so as to relieve cough.

Powder for Activating Blood Circulation, Moistening Dryness and Promoting the Production of Body Fluid (huoxue runzao shengjin tang)

Ingredients

Radix Angelicae Sinensis	10 g
Radix Paeoniae Alba	10 g
Radix Asparagi	10 g
Radix Ophiopogonis	10 g
Radix Trichosanthis	10 g
Semen Persicae	6 g

Flos Carthami	6 g
Radix Rehmanniae Praeparata	20 g

Decoct the above ingredients in a right amount of water for oral administration.

Efficacy

Nourishing blood, activating blood circulation, promoting the production of body fluid and moistening dryness; mainly for cases attributive to insufficiency of liver - blood with failure of nourishing the lung, which manifest dry and lusterless skin, constipation, emaciation, red and dry tongue, small pulse.

Indications

1. Applicable to cases with sudden loss of vision, drry and irritated eyes, dry mouth and throat, reddish and uncoated tongue with wiry and small pulse, which are attributive to the insufficiency of liver - yin and lack of blood supply of eyes.

2. For cases of retrograde menstruation manifest epistaxis, flushed cheeks, dry mouth with unwiling to drink, dry stools, reddish and uncoated tongue, wiry and small or wiry and unsmooth pulse, which are attributive to insufficiency of yin - blood, dysfunction of liver and extravasation of blood, apply *Radix Cyathulae* instead of *Ophiopogonis* to guide the blood back to the vessels.

3. Also applicable to cases of pulmonary tuberculosis, atelectasis, persistent hepatitis and cirrhosis of liver with constipation and dry skin, which attributive to insufficiency of liver - blood and failure of nourishing the lung; and to cases with embolism of central retinal artery and thrombosis of central retinal vein marked by sudden loss of vision, which are attributive to the insufficiency of yin - blood.

Interpretation

paeoniae Alba, *Angelicae Sinensis* and *Rehmanniae Praeparata* can nourish the liver - blood to prevent the attack of lung by liver - fire. *Asparagi*, *Ophiopogonis* and *Trichosanthis* can nourish lung - yin which will supply body fluid to the skin and large intestines when it is sufficient. *Semen Persicae* and *Flos Carthami* are selected with *Angelicae Sinensis* to promote blood circulation and body fluid distribution.

Powder for Antiphlogosis

(Baidu san)

Ingredients

Rhizoma seu Radix Notopterygii	12 g
Radix Angelicae Pubescentis	12 g
Radix Bupleuri	10 g
Radix Peucedani	10 g
Rhizoma Ligustici Chuanxiong	10 g
Radix Codonopsis Pilosulae	6 g
Fructus Aurantii	6 g
Poria	6 g
Radix Platycodi	6 g
Radix Glycyrrhizae	3 g
Herba Menthae	3 g
Rhizoma Zingiberis Recens	3 pcs

Decoct the above ingredients in a right amount of water for oral administration.

Efficacy

Benefiting vital qi and expelling the evils from the body surface, eliminating the wind and dampness evil; mainly for cases with insufficiency of healthy qi and attacked by exogenous wind, cold and dampness evil, which are manifested by chilliness, fever, headache, no sweating, general aching, stuffy nose, heavy voice, productive cough, whitish and greasy fur on the tongue, floating and weak pulse, etc..

Indications

1. Applicable to skin infections which are attributive to wind – cold – dampness superficies – syndrome.

2. By adding *Fructus Forsythiae* and *Flos Lonicerae*, and omitting *Codonopsis Pilosulae*, another prescription named *Powder of Forsythiae for Antiphlogosis* is formed. It is indicated for the initial stage of skin infections attributive to virulent heat evil attacking the superficies.

3. By adding *Herba Schizonepetae* and *Radix Ledebouriellae* and omitting *Codonopsis Pilosulae*, *Zingiberis Recens* and *Menthae*, another prescription named

Powder of Schizonepetae and Ledebouriellae for Antiphlogosis is formed. It is indicated for affections of exogenous wind, cold and dampness evil, which are manifested by chilliness, fever, heavy sensation of head and body, cough, heavy voice, white and greasy fur on the tongue, wiry and tense pulse, etc..

4. Also applicable to cases of influenza, emphysema complicated by infection, malaria, acute cellulitis, etc., which are attirbutive to the affection of wind, cold and dampness evil in cases of the insufficiency of healthy qi.

Interpretation

Notopterygii and *Angelicae Pubescentis* not only can disperse wind-cold evil, but also can eliminate dampness and relieve pain. The former distributes upwardly and the latter downwardly, and they act on the whole body when used together. A small amount of *Codonopsis Pilosulae* is applied together with *Bupleuri*, *Ligustici Chuanxiong*, *Zingiberis Recens* and *Menthae* to invigorate vital qi and expel the evil factors from the body surface by sweating. A small amount of *Poria* is applied together with those drugs of *Peucedani*, *Aurantii* and *Platycodi* to eliminate sputum and relieve cough. *Radix Glycyrrhizae* serves to regulate the other drugs. This prescription combines both tonics and diaphoretics together, and possesses the advantage of producing sweating but not damaging the healthy qi, and that of supporting the healthy qi but not retaining the evils.

Powder for Clearing Away Heat in Upper of Middle Jiao (Liang ge san)

Ingredients

Fructus Forsythiae	15 g
Fructus Gardeniae	6 g
Radix Scutellariae	6 g
Radix et Rhizoma Rhei	6 g
Natrii Sulfas (mixed with decoction)	6 g
Radix Glycyrrhizae Praeparata	6 g
Folium Menthae	6 g
Herba Lophatheri	3 g
Mel (mixed with decoction)	q.s.

Decoct the above ingredients in a right amount of water for oral administration.

Efficacy

Clearing away heat evil from the upper jiao and relaxing bowel movement; mainly for cases with overabundance of heat evil over the upper and middle jiao, which are manifested by fever, thirst, burning sensation over the chest, aphthae, constipation, darkish urine, or rashes due to stomach – heat, mania, red tongue with yellowish or whitish fur and rapid pulse.

Indications

1. For cases of eruptive stage of measles attributed to virulent heat, which are manifested by deep red rashes, conjunctivitis, dry nose, dyspnea, thirst with desire for drink, red tongue and rapid pulse, add *radix Arnebiae seu Lithospermi* and *Flos Carthami* to and subtract *Natrii Sulfas* from the prescription to clear away heat evil and detoxicate.

2. For cases attributed to virulent heat at qifen, which are manifested by pharyngitis, fever, thirst, red tongue with yellowish fur, add *Indigo Naturalis* and *Flos Lonicerae* to and subtract *Natrii Sulfas* and *Rhei* from the prescription to clear away the heat evil and ease the throat.

3. Applicable to cases of acute bronchitis, lobar pneumonia, lobar pneumonia, periodontitis and suppurative tonsillitis, which are attributed to overabundance of heat evil over the upper and middle jiao.

Interpretation

Forsythiae has the effect of clearing away the heat evil from the chest and is used in large dosage as the chief drug. *Gardeniae*, *Scutellariae*, *menthae* and *Lophatheri* are helpful to clear away the heat evil from the upper jiao, while *Rhei* and *Natrii Sulfas* to purge the fire evil from the middle jiao and promote the bowel movement. But for the hollow – organ sthenia – syndrome with consumption of body fluid by stomach – heat, a strong purgative is not necessary, so *Glycyrrhizae* and *Mel* are applied to decrease the purgative effect of *Natrii Sulfas* and *Rhei* which also serve to clear away the virulent heat evil, preserve the stomach fluid and moisten the dry feces. In summary, this prescription can clear away the heat evil from the upper and middle jiao with a mild purgative effect.

Powder for Expelling Five Kinds of Stagna

(Wuji san)

Ingredients

Radix Angelicae Dahuricae	10 g
Rhizoma Ligustici Chuanxiong	10 g
Poria	10 g
Radix Angelicae Sinensis	10 g
Radix Paeoniae Alba	10 g
Rhizoma Pinelliae Praeparata	10 g
Exocarpium Citri Grandis	10 g
Fructus Aurantii	10 g
Rhizoma Atractylodis	10 g
Rhizoma Zingiberis	10 g
Cortex magnoliae Officinalis	10 g
Cortex Cinnamomi	6 g
Herba Ephedrae	6 g
Radix Platycodi	6 g
Radix Glycyrrhizae Praeparata	3 g
Rhizoma Zingiberis Recens	3 pcs

Decoct the above ingredients in a right amount of water for oral administration.

Efficacy

Expelling superficial evil, warming middle jiao, regulating vital qi and blood, and dispersing phlegm; mainly for cases attributive to attack of exogenous cold to a person with interior cold, retention of phlegm – dampness and stagnation of vital qi and blood, which manifest fever, chilliness, headache, anhidrosis, rigidity of neck, abdominal distention, nausea, vomiting, increased borborygmus, loose stools, cold and pain over the abdomen.

Indications

1. Applicable to cases of dysmenorrhea with tenderness which can be relieve by warmth, oligomenorrhea, cold limbs, white and greasy fur on the tongue, sunken and

...e, which are attributive to accumulation of cold – dampness in the uterus and ...ation of vital qi and blood.

2. For cases with soft but localized masses in the abdomen, abdominal fullness and pain, accompanied with aversion to cold, fever, headache, anhidrosis, white and greasy fur on the tongue, floating and wiry, large pulse, which are attributive to the stagnation of vital qi and blood and the attack of exogenous wind – cold, add *Semen Arecase* to the prescription. For cases without the attack of exogenous wind – cold, omit *Ephedrae* and *Angelicae Dahuricae* from it.

3. Also applicable to cases of common cold of gastrointestinal type and biliary infection marked by fever, chillinessand abdominal fullness, which are attributive to attack of exogenous cold to a person with interior cold; to cases of endometritis, hysteromyoma and vegetative neurosis marked by dysmenorrhea which is attributive to attack of cold – dampness, stagnation of vital qi and blood; and to cases of congestive hepatomegaly and chronic malaria marked by abdominal mass which is attributive to stagnation of vital qi and blood.

Interpretation

Ephedrae and *Angelicae Dahuricae* are diaphoretics; *Zingiberis* and *Cortex Cinnamomi* can warm middle jiao and disperse cold. The above four drugs together serve as a remedy for various kinds of stagnation. *Atractylodis* and *Magnoliae Officinalis* can activate the spleen and dry dampness to relieve the stagnation of food. *Citri Grandis* and *Pinelliae Praeparata* can regulate vital qi and disperse phlegm to relieve the stagnation of phlegm. *Platycodi* and *Aurantii* can regulate descending and ascending of vital qi to relieve the stagnation of blood. *Glycyrrhizae* and *Zingiberis Recens* coordinate the functions of the above drugs.

Powder for Expelling Lung – Heat
(Xiebai san)

Ingredients

Cortex Lycii Radicis	30 g
Cortex Mori Radicis	30 g
Radix Glycyrrhizae Praeparata	3 g
Fructus Oryzae Sativae	20 g

Efficacy

Purging the lung - heat, relieving dyspnea and cough; mainly for cases due to consumption of yin by lung - heat, which are manifested by cough, dyspnea, feverish sensation over the skin, afternoon fever, red tongue with yellow fur, small and rapid pulse.

Indications

1. The prescription is suitable for cases in which the hidden fire is not too strong and the consumption of yin is not so severe. For cases with potent heat evil in the lung channel, add *Radix Scutellariae* or *Gypsum Fibrosum* to enhance the effect of purging lung - heat; for cases with hectic fever due to yin - deficiency, add *Herba Artemisiae Annuae* and *Carapax Trionycis* to enhance the effect of clearing away the heat evil; for cases with severe cough of dryness - heat type, add *Semen Trichosanthis* and *Bulbus Fritillariae Cirrhosae* to moisturize lung and relieve cough.

2. Also applicable to cases of bronchitis, pneumonia, bronchial asthma, Loffler's syndrome, tropical eosinophilia, etc. with dyspneic cough attributed to consumption of yin by lung - heat.

Interpretation

Mori Radicis, sweet in taste and cold in nature, has the effects of purging lung - heat, relieving dyspnea and cough; *Lycii Radicis*, also sweet in taste and cold in nature, serve to purge the fire retained in the lung. The two drugs used together in a large dosage are good for dyspneic cough due to lung - heat. *Glycyrrhizae Praeparata* and *Oryzae Sativae* have the effect of regulating the qi and yin of the lung and stomach. The four drugs used together can purge the lung - heat but does not damage the healthy vital qi.

Powder of Armeniacae Amarum and Folium Perillae
(Xing su san)

Ingredients

Semen Armeniacae Amarum	10 g
Radix Platycodi	10 g
Poria	10 g

Rhizoma Pinelliae	10 g
Fructus Aurantii	10 g
Folium Perillae	6 g
Radix Peucedani	6 g
Exocarpium Citri Grandis	6 g
Radix Glycyrrhizae	3 g
Rhizoma Zingiberis Recens	4 pcs
Fructus Ziziphi Jujubae	3 pcs

Efficacy

Eliminating coolness and dryness and releasing the stagnated lung – qi; mainly for cases attributive to attack of exogenous coolness and dryness and the stagnation of phlegm – dampness, which are manifested by chilliness, anhidrosis, mild headache, cough with thin sputum, stuffy nose, white fur on the tongue, wiry pulse.

Indications

1. For cases with scanty expectoration, omit *Pinelliae* and *Poria* from this prescription, for cases with profuse expectoration of thin sputum, increase the dosage of *Pinelliae* and *Citri Grandis*.

2. Applicable to common cold of wind – cold type, manifested by chilliness, anhidrosis, headache, stuffy nose, cough with thin sputum, white fur on the tongue, floating pulse. \ ; 3. Also applicable to cases of emphysema complicated by infection, chronic bronchitis, bronchiectasis, influenza, etc. which are attributive to damage of the lung by coolness and dryness and stagnation of phlegm – dampness.

Interpretation

Armeniacae Amarum can release and lower the lung – energy, disperse phlegm and relieve cough. Perillae has a mild diaphoretic effect and eliminates coolness and dryness from the body surface, and its acrid – warm property is counteracted by *Armeniacae Amarum*. *Platycodi* releases lung – qi and eliminates phlegm. *Peucedani* lowers down qi and phlegm, and *Aurantii* releases the stagnated qi and promotes expectoration; they act with each other to enhance the expectorant and antitussive effect of *Armeniacae Amarum*. *Pinelliae*, *Citri Grandis* and *Poria* are applied to dry the endogenous dampness, and match with the exogenous dryness eliminating action of *Armeniacae Amarum* and *Platycodi*. *Zingiberis Recens* and *Ziziphi Jujubae* serve to regulate ying and wei, enhance the effect of *Perillae*.

Powder of Astragali seu Hedysari and Carapax Trionycis (Huangqi biejia san)

Ingredients

Radix Astragali seu Hedysari	15 g
Radix Rehmanniae	15 g
Carapax Trionycis (decocted first)	20 g
Radix Asparagi	10 g
Cortex Lycii Radicis	10 g
Radix Gentianae Macrophyllae	10 g
Radix Asteris	10 g
Rhizoma Pinelliae	10 g
Rhizoma Anemarrhenae	10 g
Radix Paeoniae Alba	10 g
Cortex Mori Radicis	10 g
Radix Codonopsis Pilosulae	10 g
Radix Bupleuri	3 g
Radix Glycyrrhizae Praeparata	3 g
Radix Platycodi	3 g
Cortex Cinnamomi	2 g
Rhizoma Zingiberis Recens	3 pcs

Efficacy

Invigorating vital qi, benefiting wei, nourishing yin and clearing away heat; mainly for cases attributive to deficiency of vital qi and yin with invvolvement of yang, which manifest burning sensation over the palms, soles and chest, afternoon fever, night sweating, cough, dry thraot, poor appetite, fatigue, shortness of breath, spontaneous sweating, pale complexion, red and tender tongue with whitish fur, small and weak pulse.

Indications

Applicable to cases of ecthyma with porfuse discharge and greyish white or dark red tissue, dry throat, night sweating, emaciation, fatigue, pale complexion, tender and red tongue, small and weak pulse, which are attributive to deficiency of vital qi and yin, and accumulation of dampness and toxic material in the interior.

2. Also applicable to cases of pulmonary tuberculosis, bone tuberculosis and osteomyelitis marked by fever and night sweat, which are attributive to deficiency of vital qi and yin with involvement of yang; and to varicose veins of lower limbs and thromboangiitis obliterans marked by ulcers and necrosis, which are attributive to deficiency of vital qi and consumption of body fluid, and accumulation of dampness and toxic material in the interior.

Interpretation

Astgragali seu Hedysari, *Codonopsis Pilosulae*, *Poria*, *Cinnamomi*, *Glycyrrhizae Praeparata* have the effects of inviograting vital energy and benefiting wie. *Bupleuri* and *Platycodi* can promote the ascending of lucid – yang and enhance the effects of the above drugs. *Carapax Trionycis*, *Asparagi*, *Paeoniae Alba* and *Rehmanniae* serve to nourish yin and clear away heat. *Mori Radicis*, *Anemarrhenae*, *Gentianae Macrophyllae* and *Lycii Radicis* are applied for clearing away asthenic heat. *Asteris* and *Pinelliae* can disperse sputum and relieve cough. In sum, this prescription aims at invigorating lung – qi and clearing away asthenic heat.

Powder of Elsholtziae seu Moslae
(Xiangru san)

Ingredients

Herba Elsholtziae seu Moslae	10 g
Semen dolichoris Album (fried)	15 g
Cortex Magnoliae Officinalis (prepared with ginger)	12 g

Efficacy

Expelling the evil from the body surface, eliminating the cold, summer – heat and dampness; mainly for cases caused by affection of exogenous cold evil and endogenous dampness evil during hot summer time, which are manifested by fatigue, anhidrosis, chilliness, feeling of oppression over the chest, poor appetite, or abdominal pain and vomiting, diarrhea, white and greasy fur on the tongue, etc..

Indications

1. It may be more effective when *Herba Agastachis* or *Caulis Perillae* are added.

2. By adding *Flos Dolichoris*, *Flos Lonicerae* and *Fructus Forsythiae*, and omitting *Dolichoris Album*, another prescription named *Additional Decoction of Elsholtziae seu Moslae* is formed. It has the effects of expelling summer – heat and dampness evil and regulating middle jiao, and is indicated for the initial stage of seasonal diseases manifested by fever, chilliness, anhidrosis, headache, chest and epigastric upset, thin and greasy fur on the tongue, etc.. This prescription is applied for dampness – heat syndrome in summer time, while the original one for cold – dampness syndrome.

3. by adding *Rhizoma Coptidis* and omitting *Dolichoris Album*, another prescription named *Decoction of Coptidis and Elsholtziae seu moslae* is formed. It has the effects of expelling cold evil from the superficies and clearing away summer – heat and dampness evil from the interior, and is indicated for summer – heat diseases with stagnation of cold evil in the superficies and dampness – heat evil in the interior, which are manifested by chilliness, fever, restlessness, thirst, loose stools, yellowish and greasy fur on the tongue, etc.. The prescription is superior for severe affection of summer – heat and dampness evil in the interior.

4. Also applicable to cases of common cold and gastroenteritis in summer time, which are attributive to superficial cold and interior dampness.

Interpretation

Elsholtzia seu Moslae is the principal drug in this prescription, which is of acrid flavour, warm nature and fragrant smell. It has the effects of expelling cold evil from the body surface, also dispelling summer – heat evil and eliminating dampness evil from the middle jiao. *Magnoliae Officinalis* is of bitter flavour and warm nature, which has the effects of promoting vital qi and easing the middle jiao. *Dolichoris Album* is of sweet flavour and mild nature, which has the effect of strengthening the spleen to eliminate dampness evil. Both of these two drugs aid *Elsholtziae seu Moslae* to eliminate summer – heat and dampness evil. The prescription as a whole takes care of both the interior and the superficies. When the superficies-syndrome is relieved, the cold and heat evil will be removed, and when the circulation of vital qi is in order, vomiting and diarrhea will be relieved.

Powder of Fritillary Bulb and Snakegourd Fruit (Beimu gualou san)

Ingredients

Bulbus Fritillariae	5 g
Fructus Trichosanthis	3 g
Poria	2 g
Exocarpium Citri Reticulatae	2 g
Radix Platycodi	2 g

Efficacy

Nourishing the lung and clearing away heat, regulating qi and resolving phlegm.

Indications

Cough due to dryness of the lung marked by difficulty in expectoration, dryness of the throat, dyspnea, etc..

Chronic bronchitis marked by cough due to dryness of the lung can be treated by the modified recipe.

Interpretation

As a principal drug, *Fritillary bulb* clears away heat and nourishes the lung, resolves phlegm to arrest cough and dispels the stagnation of phlegm and qi. *Snakegourd fruit* clears away heat and moistens the dryness, regulates qi and removes phlegm, and dispels obstruction of qi in the chest, used as an assistant drug. *Root of trichosanthes* clears heat to resolve sputum, promotes the production of body fluids to moisten dryness. *Tuckahoe* strengthens the spleen and induces diuresis to inhibit phlegm-producing sources; *Tangerine peel* regulates qi to resolve phlegm, gets the qi flowing normally and phlegm cleared away; *Root of balloonflower disperses the functional disturbance of the lung – qi.*

Modern researches have proved that the recipe has the effects of dilating the bronchi, enhancing the secretion of the mucosa of the respiratory tract and the effects of eliminating phlegm and relieving inflammation.

Cautions

Flaring up deficiency – fire type due to the deficiency of kidney – yin marked by cough, dryness of throat, flushing of zygomatic region, night sweat and other symptoms should be treated with the drugs nourishing yin purging the fire other than this recipe.

Powder of Ginseng and Astragali seu hedysari
(Renshen huangqi tang)

Ingredients

Radix Codonopsis Pilosulae	15 g
Radix Astragali seu Hedysari	15 g
Radix Rehmanniae	15 g
Radix Gentianae Macrocephyllae	15 g
Cortex Lycii Radicis	15 g
Radix Asparagi	15 g
Poria	10 g
Rhizoma Anemarrhenae	10 g
Cortex Mori Radicis	10 g
Radix Paeoniae Rubra	10 g
Carapax Trionycis	20 g
Radix Platycodi	6 g
Radix Asteris	6 g
Radix Bupleuri	6 g
Rhizoma Pinelliae Praeparata	6 g
Radix Glycyrrhizae Praeparata	3 g

Efficacy

Benefiting vital qi, promoting the production of body fluid, nourishing yin, lowering fever, dispersing phlegm and stopping cough; mainly for consumptive diseases manifested by prolonged low fever, fatigue, shortness of breath, poor appetite, feverish sensation over the precordial region, soles and palms, night sweat, emaciation, pale complexion, cough with thick sputum, tender and red tongue, weak and rapid pulse, which are attributive to impairment of vital qi and yin and attack of the lung by asthenic fire.

Indications

1. Applicable to cases of pulmonary abscess manifested by cough with purulent and foul sputum, lusterless complexion, emaciation, afternoon fever, fatigue and dyspnea.

2. Also indicated for cases with hemoptysis, irritability, shortness of breath, fatigue, plae complexion, spontaneous sweating, night sweating, tender and red tongue, wiry and small pulse, which are attributive to impairment of lung－qi and attack of the lung by liver－fire.

3. Also applicable to cases of pulmonary tuberculosis and lupus pneumonia attack of the lung by asthenic fire, and cases of bronchiectasis and pulmonary congestion with hemoptysis attributive to impairment of lung－qi and attack of the lung by liver－fire.

Interpretation

Codonopsis Pilosulae and *Astragali seu Hedysari* have the effects of benefiting vital qi and promoting the production of body fluid. *Asparagi* and *Rehmanniae* serve to nourish yin and clearing away heat. *Gentianae Macrophyllae*, *Lycii Radicis*, *Mori Radicis*, *Carapax Trionycis*, *Paeoniae Rubra*, *Anemarrhenae* and *Bupleuri* can clear away the astehnic heat of yinfen. *Asteris*, *Platycodi*, *Poria* and *Pinelliae Praeparata* are applied for expectorant and antitussive. The dry, hot and fluid－consuming effect of *Pinelliae* is inhibited by *Rehmanniae*, and the indigestable effect of the latter is counteracted by the former. *Glycyrrhizae* used together with *Codonopsis Pilosulae* and *Astragali seu Hedysari* serves to benefit vital qi and promote the production of body fluid.

Powder of Inulae
(Jinfeicao san)

Ingredients

Herba Inulae	12 g
Radix Peucedani	10 g
Rhizoma Pinelliae	10 g
Poria	10 g
Herba Asari	3 g
Radix Glycyrrhizae	3 g
Herba Schizonepetae	6 g
Rhizoma Zingiberis Recens	5 pcs
Fructus Ziziphi Jujubae	3 pcs

Efficacy

Expelling cold from the body surface, dispersing phlegm and relieving cough; mainly for cases attributive to attack of exogenous wind and cold and retention of phlegm, which manifest chilliness, fever, headache, stuffy nose, cough with profuse thin expectoration, shortness of breath, white and smooth fur on the tongue, floating and tense pulse.

Indications

1. Applicable to cases of cough with thin and whitish expectoration, which are attributive to retention of phlegm althouth without the attack of exogenous wind - cold.

2. Also applicable to common cold, acute bronchitis and emphysema complicated by pulmonary infection, which are attributive to the attack of exogenous wind - cold and retention of phlegm.

Interpretation

Inulae can eliminate the superficial pathogens from the body surface, relieve cough, disperse phlegm and expel dampness. *Schizonepetae* and *Asari* serve to expel wind - cold through the superficies when they are used together with *Inulae*. *Pinelliae*, *Zingiberis Recens* and *Poria*, used together with *Inulae* and *Asari*, can promote diuresis, disperse phlegm and relieve cough. *Peucedani* is good for lowering the adverse rising qi, but it can disperse phlegm and relieve cough when it is used together with *Zingiberis Recens*. *Asari*, *Jujubae* and *Glycyrrhizae*, when used together with *Zingiberis Recens*, can regulate ying and wei and eliminate the superficial pathogens. In sum, this prescription aims chiefly at the disorders of the interior by dispersing phlegm and relieving cough and also at those of the superficies by eliminating dampness and other pathogens.

Powder of Ledebouriellae for Dispersing the Superficies (Fangfeng tongsheng san)

Ingredients

Radix Ledebouriellae	10 g
Fructus Forsythiae	10 g
Fructus Gardeniae	10 g
Herba Schizonepetae	6 g
Herba Ephedrae	6 g
Rhizoma Ligustici Chuanxiong	6 g
Radix Angelicae Sinensis	6 g
Radix Paeoniae Alba	6 g
Rhizoma Atractylodis Macrocephalae	6 g
Radix et Rhizoma Rhei	6 g
Natrii Sulfas	6 g
Radix Scutellariae	6 g
Talcum	20 g
Gypsum Fibrosum	15 g
Herba Menthae	3 g
Radix Platycodi	3 g
Radix Glycyrrhizae	3 g
Rhizoma Zingiberis Recens	3 pcs

Decoct the above ingredients in a right amount of water for oral administration.

Efficacy

Expelling wind from the body surface, clearing away heat and promoting bowel movement; mainly for sthenia – syndrome of both the superficies and the interior after the attack of exogenous wind – heat and the retention of heat in the interior, which is manifested by aversion to cold, fever, dizziness, bitter and dry mouth, conjunctivitis, sore – throat, feeling of oppression over the chest, constipation, dysuria with reddish urine, red tongue with white or yellow fur, floating and smooth, rapid pulse.

Indications

1. Applicable to cases of early stage of superficial pyogenic infection with local signs of inflammation, chilliness, fever, bitter mouth, constipation, oliguria, red tongue with white fur, floating and rapid pulse.

2. Also indicated for cases of urticaria and eczema with thin and white fur on the tongue, floating and rapid pulse, which are attributive to simultaneous existence of sthenia - syndrome in the superficies and the interior.

3. Also applicable to cases of influenza, poliomyelitis, infectious mononucleosis, mumps, acute cellulitis, erysipelas, acute lymphangitis, etc., which are attributive to simultaneous existence of sthenia - syndrome in the superficies and the interior after attack of exogenous wind - heat and retention of heat in the body.

Interpretation

Ledebouriellae, *Schizonepetae*, *Ephedrae*, *Zingiberis Recens* and *Menthae* serve to expel wind by sweating. *Rhei* and *Natrii Sulfas* eliminate the internal heat by purgation, and *Gardeniae* and *Talcum* clear away heat by diuresis. *Platycodi*, *Gypsum Fibrosum*, *Scutellariae* and *Forsythiae* can clear away heat from the lung and stomach. All the above drugs act together to eliminate heat from the upper and the lower part of the body, and treat both the superficies and the interior syndrome. *Angelicae Sinensis*, *Ligustici Chuanxiong* and *Paeoniae Alba* have the effects of expelling wind and nourishing blood, and *Atractylodis Macrocephalae* and *Glycyrrhizae* serve to strengthen the spleen and regulating the stomach; they cooperate each other to exert a diaphoretic effect without damaging the superficies, and exert a purgative effect without impairing the interior. In sum, this prescription involves the therapeutic principles of diaphoretic, heat - eliminating, purgative and tonifying simultaneously, aiming at clearing away the internal heat chiefly. The application of *Natrii Sulfas* and *Rhei* is for purging heat.

Powder of Lonicerae and Forsythiae
(yinqiao san)

Ingredients

Flos Lonicerae	12 g
Fructus Forsythiae	12 g

Fructus Arctii	10 g
Semen Sojae Praeparatum	10 g
Rhizoma Phragmitis	10 g
Radix Platycodi	5 g
Herba Menthae	5 g
Herba Lophatheri	5 g
Radix Glycyrrhizae	5 g
Spica Schizonepetae	5 g

Efficacy

Expelling wind and heat evil, clearing away heat evil and toxic material; mainly for cases due to exogenous wind and heat evil, which are manifested by fever, mild chilliness, sore-throat, headache, thirst, red tip of the tongue with thin white fur or thin yellowish fur, floating and rapid pulse, etc..

Indications

1. The therapeutic principle of this prescription is reasonable, the concept of compatibility is strict and its curative effect is fruitful, and has become a typical recipe for common cold of wind-heat type. For cases with extreme thirst, add *Radix Trichosanthis* to promote the production of saliva and quench thirst; for cases with sore-throat, add *Radix Scrophulariae* to clear away the heat evil and ease the throat.

2. For the initial stage of measles attributive to stagnation of wind and heat evil in the superficies, which is manifested by fever, thirst and incomplete eruption, add *Radix Puerariae* to let out the eruptions.

3. For cases at the onset of skin infections attributive to super ficies-syndrome of wind-heat type, add *Herba Taraxaci* or *Folium Isatidis* to clear away heat evil and toxic material, and dispersing the accumulation of evils.

4. Also applicable to cases of acute tonsillitis, influenza, mumps, measles, encephalitis B epidemic meningitis and acute suppurative infection, which are attributive to wind-heat syndrome of the superficies.

Interpretation

Lonicerae and *Forsythiae* are selected as principal drugs which have mild action to let the evil out of the body and clear away heat evil and toxic material, so as to prevent the evil from attacking the interior. *Schizonepetae*, *Menthae* and *Sojae Praeparatum* can expel the evils from the surface of the body owing to their acrid flavour. *Arctii*, *Platycodi* and *Glycyrrhizae* have the effects of clearing away heat evil and toxic material to ease the throat. *Lophatheri* and *Phragmitis* have the effects of clearing away heat evil and promoting the production of body fluid to relieve thirst. This prescription constitutes an acrid – cool remedy by combining the drugs of clearing away heat evil and toxic material with those of expelling the evil from the body surface. This model of compatibility exerts a great influence upon the later generation, and many new set prescriptions for common cold are composed of its modifications.

Powder of phellodendri and Atractylodis
(Ermiao san)

Ingredients

Cortex Phellodendri	2 g
Rhizoma Atractylodis	12 g.

Efficacy

Clearing away heat and drying dampness; mainly for cases with redness, swelling pain and increased temperature over the knees and legs, oliguria with yellow urine, yellow and greasy fur on the tongue, which are attributive to downward attack of dampness – heat.

Indications

1. Cases of discharge, itching of the vulva, red tongue with yellow and greasy fur, smooth and rapid pulse, which are attributive to downward attack of dampness – heat evil.

2. Also applicable to cases of rheumatic arthritis, gouty arthritis, mycotic vaginitis and cervicitis attributive to downward attack of dampness – heat.

Interpretation

Phellodendri can clear away heat by its bitter – cold nature, and *Atractylodis* dry dampness by its bitter – warm property. Because heat is a pathogen of yang nature, it must be eliminated with bitter – cold drugs.

Powder of Ten Drug's Ashes
(Shihui san)

Ingredients

Herba seu Radix Cirsii Japonici
Herba Cephalanoploris
Folium Nelumbinis
Cacumen Biotae
Rhizoma Imperatae
Radix Rubiae
Fructus Gardeniae
Radix et Rhizoma Rhei
Cortex Moutan Radicis
Cortex Trachycarpi
Succus Rhizoma Lotus
Succus Raphani q.s.

Efficacy

Cooling blood and stopping bleeding; mainly for hemorrhages due to blood – heat, esp. those from the upper parts of the body such as hematemesis, epistaxis, hemoptysis, etc. resulting from upward rushing of vital qi and fire.

Indications

1. This prescription has been widely applied for various kinds of hemorrhage with heat – syndrome as a symptomatic remedy, and the treatment for the causative condition should be carried on when the bleeding is stopped.

2. Also applicable to cases of hemoptysis and hematemesis attributive to blood – heat, occuring in bronchiectasis, pulmonary tuberculosis, pulmonary congestion, esophageal or fundal varicose, duodenal ulcer, etc..

Interpretation

Cirsii Japonici, *Cephalanoploris*, *Folium Nelumbinis*, *Cacumen Biotae* and *Imperatae*, *Rubiae* act as blood – cooling and hemostatic agents. *Gardeniae* is for clearing away heat evil and purging fire evil; *Rhei* for letting the heat downward, and both are helpful to enhance the blood – cooling effect and to stop the bleeding from the upper part. *Trachycarpi* acts as an astringent and hemostatic, and *Moutan Radicis* and *Succus Lotus* combined with *Rhei* serve to prevent the over action of astrigents which may lead to retention of blood stasis. *Succus Raphani* leads the vital qi downwards and promotes digestion, so as to enhance the heat – descending effect. As a whole, the chief action of the prescription is blood – cooling, and astringent and circulation activating as well.

Prescription for General Severe Arthralgia

Ingredients

Cortex Phellodendri	12 g
Rhizoma Atractylodis	12 g
Rhizoma Arisaematis	12 g
Ramulus Cinnamomi	6 g
Radix Clematidis	6 g
Flos Carthami	6 g
Radix Gentianae	6 g
Rhizoma Ligustici Chuanxiong	6 g
Massa Fermentata Medicinalis	6 g
Rhizoma seu Radix Notopterygii	10 g
Radix Stephaniae Tetrandrae	10 g
Radix Angelicae Dahuricae	10 g
Semen Persicae	10 g

Decoct the above ingredients in a right amount of water for oral administration.

Efficacy

Expelling wind and dampness, activating blood ciruclation, drying phlegm, clearing away heat and promoting diuresis; mainly for cases with severe and general arthralgia, limited mobility of joints, dimmish tongue with yellow and greasy fur, wiry pulse, which are attributive to attack of wind – dampness to the joint, and phlegm – heat to the meridians.

Indications

1. Applicable to cases of leucorrhagia with reddish, thick and foul discharge, pruritus of external genitalia, dimmish tongue with yellow and greasy fur, wiry and smooth pulse, which are attributive to accumulation of blood stasis and heat and downward attack of phlegm – dampness.

2. Also indicated for cases of sinusitis manifested by headache, stuffy nose, thick, purulent and foul nasal discharge, dark reddish tongue with yellow and turbid fur, wiry and smooth pulse, which are attributive to attack of the nose by phlegm – dampness and accumulation of blood stasis and heat.

3. Also applicable to cases of rheumatic arthritis and gouty arthritis attributive to the attack of wind – dampness and accumulation of phlegm – heat; to cases of senile vaginitis and submucous myoma of cervix attributive to accumulation of blood stasis and heat and downward attack of phlegm – dampness.

Interpretation

Angelicae Dahuricae is applied for eliminating wind – dampness in the face and head, *Ramulus Cinnamomi* and *Clematidis* for that in the arms and legs, and *Notopterygii* for that in the joints. *Arisaematis* and *Massa Fermentata Medicinalis* serve to dry dampness and eliminate wind. *Persicae*, *Carthami* and *Ligustici Chuanxiong* can activate blood circulation and eliminate blood stasis. *Phellodendri*, *Atractylodis*, *Stephaniae Tetrandrae* and *Gentianae* have the effects of clearing away heat and discharging dampness. In sum, the prescription can eliminate wind and dampness from the upper part of the body, activate blood circulation and dry dampness from the middle part, promote diuresis and clear away heat from the lower part.

Prescription for Treating Hemoptysis
(Kexie fang)

Ingredients

Indigo Naturalis 6 g

Semen Trichosanthis	12 g
Pumex	12 g
Fructus Gardeniae	9 g
Fructus Chebulae	6 g
Mel	q.s.
Succus Zingiberis Recens	q.s.

Decoct the above ingredients in a right amount of water for oral administration.

Efficacy

Cooling the liver, stopping bleeding, dispersing phlegm and relieving cough; mainly for cases with hemoptysis attributive to attack of liver - fire to the lung, which are manifested by cough, difficult expectoration of thick and bloody sputum, vexation, thirst, flushed cheeks, constipation, yellow fur on the tongue, wiry and rapid pulse.

Indications

1. Applicable to cases of rosacea accompanied with irritability, yellow fur, wiry and rapid pulse, which are attributive to attack of the lung by liver - fire and abnormal rising of blood, omit *Chebulae*, *Pumex* and add *Herba Artemisiae Annuae* and *Cortex Moutan Radicis*.

3. Also applicable to cases of bronchiectasis, pulmonary tuberculosis, pulmonary hypertension, etc. with hemoptysis, which are attributive to damage of the lung by liver - fire; or cases of hypertension and substitutive menstruation with epistaxis, which are attributive to hyperactivity of liver - fire and abnormal rising of blood.

Interpretation

Indigo Naturalis is applied for clearing away sthenic heat from the liver channel, cooling blood and stopping bleeding. *Gardeniae* has the effects of clearing away heart - fire, calming blood flow, and helps *Indigo Naturalis* to clear away fire stagnated in the liver channel. *Pumex* and *Trichosanthis* clear away lung - heat, disperse phlegm, moisten the lung and relieve cough. *Semen Trichosanthis* acting with *Mel* can lubricate the intestines and promote bowel movement. *Pumex* and *Succus Zingiberis* used together can enhance the expectorant effect. *Chebulae* serves to astringe the lung - qi, and also enhance the antitussive effect of the above drugs. In sum, prescription aims chiefly at clearing away liver－fire, so as to ease the lung and stop hemoptysis.

Qiongyu Extractum
(Qiongyu gao)

Ingredients

Radix Ginseng Korea	4 g
Radix Rehmanniae	32 g
Poria	8 g
Mel	20 g

Efficacy

Tonifying kidney－yin and moisturizing lung－dryness; mainly for consumptive diseases attributive to deficiency of lung－yin and kidney－yin, which manifest dry cough, dry throat, emaciation, flushed cheeks, dizzinss, tinnitus, weakness of the lower extremities, shortness of breath, spontaneous sweating, reddish uncoated tongue or crimson dry tongue, small and weak pulse.

Indications

1. Applicable to cases with hemoptysis, dryness of throat and nose, feverish sensation of face, vexation, tender red and uncoated or crimson and dry tongue, which are attributive to deficiency of lung－yin and kidney－yin and flaming up of asthenic fire.

2. Also indicated for cases with aphonia, dry throat, insomnia, feverish sensation over the palms and soles, red and uncaoted tongue, small and rapid weak pulse, which are attributive to deficiency of lung－yin and kidney－yin.

3. Also applicable to cases of tuberculosis of pharynx or larynx, chronic bronchitis, pulmonary tuberculosis, bronchiectasis and chronic laryngitis, which are attributive to deficiency of lung－yin and kidney－yin.

Interpretation

Rehmanniae is used for nourishing kidney－fluid, and *Mel* for moisturizing lung－dryness, this is the application of the principle of generation between metal (lung) and water (kidney). *Ginseng* and *Poria* can benefit vital qi and invigorate the spleen so as to support the lung. In this prescription, a large dosage of *Rehmanniae* is applied for increasing the production of fluid to suppress fire, and *Ginseng* of superior grade for benefiting vital qi and promoting the production of body fluid to relieve lung disorders.

Shenzhu Powder
(Shen zhu san)

Ingredients

Rhizoma Atractylodis	12 g
Cortex Magnoliae Officinalis	12 g
Exocarpium Citri Grandis	10 g
Herba Agastachis	10 g
Fructus Amomi	6 g
Radix Glycyrrhizae Praeparata	3 g

Efficacy

Expelling the dirty and turbid pathogens, drying dampness, activating the spleen, promoting the circulation of vital qi and regulating the function of stomach; mainly for cases attributive to the attack of dirty and turbid pathogens, which manifest fever, chilliness, feeling of oppression over the chest, abdominal pain and fullness, nausea, vomiting, diarrhea, white and greasy fur on the tongue, floating and slow pulse.

Indications

1. For cases of sinusitis with nasal discharge, headache, stuffy nose, dizziness, white and smooth fur on the tongue, soft and floating, slow pulse, which are attributed to the attack of dampness to the upper orifice.

2. Also applicable to common cold of gastrointestinal type and acute gastroenteritis, which are attributive to the attack of dirty and turbid pathogens.

Interpretation

Agastachis can expel the dirty pathogens and stop vomiting. *Magnoliae Officinalis* has the effects of promoting vital qi circulation, soothing the chest and relieving fullness. *Citri Grandis* can regulate vital qi, dry dampness and ease the middle jiao. *Amomi* is used for strengthening the function of the spleen to stop vomiting. *Atractylodis* can expel the pathogens from the superficies and eliminate dampness when it is used together with *Agastachis*. When it combines with *Magnoliae Officinalis*, *Citri Grandis* and *Glycyrrhizae Praeparata*, the *Powder for Regulating the Function of Stomach* is formed, which can dry dampness, strengthen the spleen, promote the circulation of vital qi and soothe the stomach. Most of the drugs in this prescription, except *Glycyrrhizae*, are acrid and fragrant agents which can expel the dirty pathogens and disperse dampness.

Small Blue Dragon Decoction
(Xiaoqinglong tang)

Ingredients

Herba Ephedrae	10 g
Radix Paeoniae Alba	10 g
Ramulus Cinnamomi	10 g
Rhizoma Pinelliae Praeparata	10 g
Rhizoma Zingiberis	5 g
Fructus Schisandrae	5 g
Herba Asari	3 g
Radix Glycyrrhizae Praeparata	3 g

Decoct the above ingredients in a right amount of water for oral administration.

Efficacy

Expelling exogenous evil from the body surface, dispersing cold evil, warming the lung and eliminating the phlegm retention; mainly for cases attributive to the attack of exogenous wind, cold evil and the retention of water, manifested by chilliness, fever, anhidrosis, dyspneic cough with thin sputum, or general edema, pale tongue with whitish and greasy fur.

Indications

1. This prescription is not the remedy specified for the exogenous cold – syndrome

with retention of phlegm in the interior. It may also be applied for those cases with cough and expectoration of thin, whitish frothy sputum, signifying retention of phlegm in the interior although the exogenous cold evil is absent. *Ephedrae* should be prepared with honey in this case to open the inhibited lung – qi and relieving cough.

2. Applicable to cases of diffused fluid – retention complicated by the attack of superficies by wind – coldd evil, manifested by general edema, heavy sensation of body, chilliness, anhidrosis, productive cough with white and frothy sputum, white fur, wiry and tense pulse.

3. By adding *Gypsum Fibrosum* to this prescription, it is named *Small Blue Dragon Decoction with Gypsum Fibrosum*. Its indications are the same as those of *Small blue Dragon Decoction* accompanied with interior – heat syndrome.

4. Also applicable to cases of bronchial asthma, senile emphysema and chronic bronchitis marked by dyspneic cough, which are attributive to retention of phlegm complicated by exogenous cold – syndrome.

Interpretation

Ephedrae has the effects of expelling the exogenous evil from the body surface, dispersing cold evil, relieving asthma and cough. *Ramulus Cinnamomi* can warm the lung to eliminate the phlegm retention besides helping the effect of *Ephedrae*. *Zingiberis* and *Asari* have the effects of expelling exogenous wind – cold evil and warming the spleen to eliminate the phlegm retention in the interior when they are used together with *Cinnamomi*. *Pinelliae Praeparata* can dry the dampness to eliminate the phlegm. *Schisandrae* can warm the lung and preserve vital qi to prevent the exhaustion of lung – qi. *Paeoniae Alba* combined with *Cinnamomi* is used to regulate ying – qi and wei – qi and expel the cold evil from the muscles. *Glycyrrhizae Praeparata* helps *Cinnamomi* to warm the spleen and eliminate the retention of phlegm. In sum, the prescription is chiefly used for the interior – syndrome (warming the lung to eliminate the phlegm retention).

Sweet Wormwood and Turtle Shell Decoction
(Qinghao biejia tang)

Ingredients

Herba Artemisiae	6 g
Carapax Trionycis	15 g

Radix Rehmanniae	12 g
Rhizoma Anemarrhenae	6 g
Cortex Moutan Radicis	9 g

Decoct the above ingredients in a right amount of water for oral administration.

Efficacy

Nourishing yin and expelling pathogenic heat from the interior.

Indications

Latent heat in the interior of the body, manifested by fever at night and normal in the morning, absence of perspiration after fever subsides, polyphagia with emaciation, reddened tongue with little coating and rapid pulse.

The recipe is modified to deal with such diseases as pulmonary tuberculosis and other chronic consumptive diseases related to hyperactivity of fire due to yin deficiency.

Interpretation

In the recipe, ***Fresh – water turtle shell*** directly enters the yin system and, being salty in taste and cold in nature, has the effect of nourishing yin so as to reduce fever of deficiency type; ***Sweet wormwood*** is used as an aromatic with the function of clearing heat from the channels and making it off from the body. Both the above ingredients are principal drugs and the combined application of the two yields the effect of expelling heat without injuring yin while replenishing yin with no influence on the expulsion of pathogens. ***Dried rehmannia root***, an ingredient with a sweet taste and cool nature, and ***Wind – weed*** which is bitter, cold and moist, both strengthen the efficacy of ***Fresh – water turtle shell*** in reducing fever of deficiency type. ***Moutan bark*** has the effect of cooling the blood and removing heat from the body and is used to assist ***Sweet wormwood*** in removing latent heat in the yin system.

Modern researches have confirmed that the recipe possesses the efficacy in tranquilizing the mind, relieving inflammation, resisting bacteria, inhibiting hyperfunction of catabolism, nourishing the body and consolidating the constitution.

Cautions

1. As *Sweet wormwood* in the above recipe is not resistant to high temperature, it should not be decocted for too long. It may be infused in boiling water for oral administration.

2. It is not advisable for cases with tendency to convulsion due to yin – deficiency.

Two Old Drugs Decoction
(Erchen tang)

Ingredients

Rhizoma Pinelliae	15 g
Pericarpium Citri Reticulatae	15 g
Poria	9 g
Radix Glycyrrhizae Praeparata	3 g

Add 3 grams of *fresh ginger* and a piece of *black plum* into the above recipe. Decoct the above ingredients in a right amount of water for oral administration.

Efficacy

Removing dampness to resolve phlegm, and regulating the stomach. Dampness – phlegm syndrome marked by cough with profuse whitish sputum, fullness sensation in the chest, nausea, vomiting, dizziness, palpitation, whitish and moist fur of the tongue and slippery pulse.

Indications

Bronchitis, gastritis, catarrhal gastritis and other diseases marked by dampness – phlegm syndrome can be treated by the modified recipe.

The recipe belongs to pungent and drying prescriptions, therefore, it is contraindicated in patients suffering from pulmonary tuberculosis with hemoptysis, sticky phlegm due to deficiency of yin and bloody phlegm.

Interpretation

Pinellia tuber, with a pungent flavor and warm and dry nature, is effective in removing dampness to resolve phlegm and lowering the adverse flow of qi and regulating the stomach to arrest vomiting, as a principal drug. *Tangerine peel* as an assistant drug, with the effect of regulating qi to remove dampness, enables the spleen and eliminates dampness; *fresh ginger*, being able to lower the adverse flow of qi and resolve phlegm, can not only reduce the toxic effect of *Rhizoma Pinelliae* but also strengthen the effects of promoting qi – flow and resolving phlegm of *Pinellia tuber* and *Tangerine peel*. A small amount of *black plum* astringes the lung – qi. The three drugs above are used as adjuvent drugs. *Prepared licorice root*, as a guiding drug, coordinates the effects of the other drugs, moistens the lung and regulates the stomach.

Modern reasearches have proved that the recipe has the effects of strengthening the stomach to arrest vomiting, eliminating phlegm to relieve cough and preventing and treating ulcers.

Zaizao Powder
(Zaizao san)

Ingredients

Radix Astragali seu Hedysari	12 g
Radix codonopsis Pilosulae	10 g
Ramulus Cinnamomi	6 g
Radix Paeoniae Alba	6 g
Radix Aconiti Praeparata	6 g
Rhizoma seu Radix Notopterygii	6 g
Radix Ledebouriellae	6 g
Rhizoma Ligustici Chuanxiong	6 g
Herba Asari	3 g
Radix Glycyrrhizae Praeparata	3 g
Rhizoma Zingiberis Recens	5 pcs
Fructus Ziziphi Jujubae	2 pcs0

Efficacy

Supporting yang – qi to promote sweating, benefiting vital qi and expelling superficial evils from body surface; mainly for cases of common cold of wind – cold type with a yang – deficiency constitution, manifested by fever with predominant chilliness, headache, rigidity of neck, anhidrosis, cold limbs, tiredness, pale complexion, low voice, pale tongue with whitish fur, sunken and weak pulse or floating and large, weak pulse, etc..

Indications

1. Applicable to the early stage of pyogenic infection of skin, manifested by local swelling and pain but no erythema nor heat, with predominant fever, chilliness, anhidrosis, cold limbs, no thirst, thin and whitish fur on the tongue, floating and large, weak pulse, which are attributive to attack of exogenous wind – cold and deficiency of yang – qi in the body.

2. Also indicated for cases of arthralgia with wandering pain, chilliness, fever, anhidrosis, cold limbs, tiredness, flat taste of the mouth, floating and large, weak pulse, which are attributive to attack of wind – cold – dampness evil to a person with yang – deficiency constitution.

3. Also applicable to cases of upper respiratory infection, mumps, rheumatic fever, rheumatoid arthritis, carbuncle, furuncle, acute cellulitis, etc., marked by chilliness and fever, which are attributive to deficiency of yang – qi and the attack of exogenous wind – cold – dampness or wind – cold evil.

Interpretation

This prescription is characterized by simultaneous application of cold – expelling and yang – supporting drugs. *Ramulus cinnamomi*, *Notopterygii*, *Ledebouriellae*, *Asari*, *Ligustici Chuanxiong* and *Zingiberis Recens* are diaphoretics for expelling cold. If only diaphoretics are used for those cases with a yang – deficiency constitution, not only perspiration does not occur but also the deficiency of yang would be aggravated, or even yang exhaustion after profuse sweating may ensue. So *Astragali seu Hedysari* and *Codonopsis* are applied to benefit yang – qi, and *Aconiti* is helpful for strengthen yang and promoting sweating. *Paeoniae Alba* and *Ziziphi Jujubae* can nourish blood. When used together with *Astragali seu Hedysari*, *Paeoniae Alba* exerts an astringent effect to prevent over sweating.

Zuogui Decoction
(Zuogui yin)

Ingredients

Radix Rehmanniae Praeparata 20 g
Fructus Corni 10 g
Rhizoma Dioscoreae 10 g
Fructus Lycii 10 g
Poria 6 g
Radix Glycyrrhizae Praeparata 3 g

Decoct the above ingredients in a right amount of water for oral administration.

Efficacy

Nourishing kidney – yin; mainly for cases attributive to insufficiency of kidney – yin, manifested by lumbago, nocturnal emission, night sweat, dry throat, dizziness, reddish tongue, slow and rapid pulse.

Indications

The chief action of this prescription is to nourish kidney – yin, for cases with dry throat attributive to the inability to generate each other between the lung and the kidney, add *Radix Ophiopogonis* to nourish lung – yin; for cases with hectic fever and profuse sweating attributive to yin – deficiency and fire hyperactivity, add *Cortex Lycii Radicis* to clear away the astehnic heat.

2. Also applicable to cases of tuberculosis, hypertension, hypothyroidism, *Addison's disease, etc. which are attributive to insufficiency of kidney – yin but without hyperactivity of fire.*

Interpretation

Rehmanniae Praeparata tonifies kidney – yin, *Corni* nourishes liver – yin, and *Dioscoreae* invigorates spleen – yin. This prescription tonifies three yin at the same time, similar to the *Bolus of Six Drugs Containing Rehmanniae Praeparata*. But the latter deals with the cases with deficiency of yin and hyperactivity of fire, while the *Zuogui Decoction* is indicated for yin – deficiency cases without hyperactivity of fire. So *Lycii* is applied in the prescription for tonifying yin – blood, and a small dosage of *Poria* and *Glycyrrhizae Praeparata* for strengthening the spleen and benefiting vital qi.

图书在版编目(CIP)数据

中医治疗呼吸系统疾病:英文./侯景伦,周训梅主编.
—北京:学苑出版社,1996.8
ISBN7—5077—1205—2

Ⅰ.中… Ⅱ.①侯… ②周… Ⅲ.①呼吸系统疾病—中医治疗法—英文 Ⅳ.R.259.6

中国版本图书馆 CIP 数据核字(96)第 13295 号

中医治疗呼吸系统疾病

主编 侯景伦 周训梅

编委 赵 昕 李国华 耿春娥

学苑出版社出版
(中国北京万寿路西街 11 号)
邮政编码 100036
北京大兴沙窝店印刷厂印刷
中国国际图书贸易总公司发行
(中国北京车公庄西路 35 号)
北京邮政信箱第 399 号 邮政编码 100044
英文版 16 开本
1996 年 8 月第一版第一印刷
ISBN7—5077—1205—2/R·215

08700
14—E—3049P